Arthritis

YOUR QUESTIONS ANSWERED

Arthritis

YOUR QUESTIONS ANSWERED

Dr Charles Dobrée

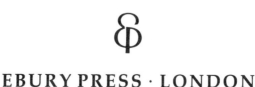

EBURY PRESS · LONDON

Published by Ebury Press
Division of The National Magazine Company Ltd
Colquhoun House
27-37 Broadwick Street
London W1V 1FR

First impression 1988
Copyright © 1988 Charles Dobrée

ISBN 0 85223 603 4

Senior Editor: Fiona MacIntyre
Editor : Miren Lopategui
Designer: Gwyn Lewis

Typeset by Text Filmsetters Ltd, London
Printed and bound in Great Britain at
The Bath Press, Avon

Contents

Notes: It must be emphasized that this book is intended merely as a general guide to the subject of arthritis, and is in no way intended to be a substitute for professional medical advice. When in doubt, therefore, *always* consult your doctor.

Throughout this book, for 'he' read 'he or she'.

General Introduction

I expect that, like me, when the title of a book has attracted your attention, the first question that passes through your mind as you pick it up and flip through it is, what sort of book is this? From the title, it's a subject that interests you, but, you ask yourself, is it a book for me?

Well, I hope that it *is* a book for you because in my experience as a doctor asking questions is of fundamental importance. I hope that, in the following pages, your questions about arthritis will be answered.

This book is all about answering your questions. Right from the start, we're going to adopt that format. You will see your questions in italics and will find my answers underneath them.

So, let's get cracking. What's the first question?

What's this book about?

This book is about helping you understand all aspects of arthritis. It is a book with an emphasis on the various treatments available – both orthodox and those that come under the description of 'alternative'. But it also takes into account the fact that treatment in itself can sometimes be of little value if it is not seen in conjunction with other forms of help. And that such help – as, for example, in the form of mechanical aids – can be more trouble than it is worth if it is either used incorrectly or is unsuited to the environment that it is placed in. I have therefore emphasized ways in which you can alter your environment to your best advantage without having to spend a fortune.

In other words, this book is a practical guide designed to help all those with arthritis to adapt more easily to their various degrees of handicap.

Does the book go into the medical causes of the various types of arthritis?

Yes, I also deal with these aspects. I realize that most people are now much more aware than they ever were about the nature and cause of disease. However, I also appreciate, from talking to patients, that there are various levels of understanding.

Therefore, what I have done at the start of the book, is to explain in simple terms what is meant by arthritis. Then, I have included a more detailed look at the various forms of arthritis and related diseases, and, finally, for those readers who want further information, I have included two glossaries (pp.139-145). The first of these deals with the various drugs used in treatment and also goes into the problems sometimes encountered with their use. The second covers some of the complex terminology that you may come across. Many of the terms in this glossary have not been used in this book but I have included them in case you have come across them either in conversations with your doctor or in other books.

But can't my doctor answer these questions?

Yes, he can answer these questions and I would not, for one moment, try to take your doctor's place. In fact, you will find, throughout the book, that I advise you to go to your doctor whenever you are in any doubt about any points that seem unclear, or if you want his clarification and balanced opinion about controversial treatments. But we live in an imperfect world and I, as a doctor, am only all too well aware of the limited time that I have available to explain fully to my patients what their problem is and how I propose to treat it.

· But shouldn't my doctor find time to explain fully to me what precisely my problem is?

Yes, of course. But I know from my own experience that there just isn't the time. There should be but there never is. It is precisely because of this limitation of time that I decided to write this book. Because, over the years, it has become clear to me that there are a number of questions about arthritis that patients want answered.

I have collected many of these questions together and, at my desk, have imagined that you are sitting opposite me and that we are having a consultation. The nice thing about it is that we both know that there isn't a full waiting room, with other patients clamouring to get in and that we are not going to be interrupted by the telephone. We are under no pressure to have to complete the consultation in a certain period of time and know that we can break off our conversation when we feel like it and take it up again, at our leisure.

Will I be able to understand the medical terminology?

Don't worry about complicated medical words. One of the basic things that I have set out to do is to avoid using confusing or complicated terminology. In fact, I hope that you will forgive me, in some instances, if I appear to be explaining the obvious. It is just that experience with patients has taught me that one of the major stumbling blocks in communication between doctor and patient is invariably the assumption on the doctor's part that the patient automatically understands him. Often, a patient is too polite or feels that he should not pursue a particular point because he doesn't like to interrupt his doctor, to ask him to explain, in simple terms, just exactly what he means. And this is where the problems start. Once misunderstanding arises, communication begins to break down and may never fully be rebuilt.

What sort of things will you be discussing?

I shall be clearly defining the specific medical problems that are, by tradition, thought of as being arthritic in nature. In so doing I shall hope, on the one hand, to dispel many commonly held myths and, on the other, to try and explain, in simple yet helpful terms, the true nature of the various accompanying diseases that are encountered in arthritis.

Is this book only for people with arthritis?

No, because I decided, when setting out to write this book, that it would be best to inform as many people as possible about the problem. There are a great deal of popular misconceptions about what really constitutes arthritic disease and I want to put all such problems in a context where they can be rationally understood because public education, in this field, is important.

But you are quite right to ask this question because if you do not suffer from arthritis yourself there will be parts of this book that will not concern you directly, but which will nevertheless, I am sure, be of interest to you.

One piece of advice that I would give you, right from the start, is to skip through the book, decide upon those parts of it that concern you directly and then, if you want to, read those sections that interest you, even though they might not have anything to do with your specific problem. Some people will not have any of the problems listed in this book. But this book is also written for such people. At first sight, this may seem strange. But one of the themes that I emphasize throughout the book is that not only is it important for the person with the problem to have a better understanding of his or her disease, it is equally important for the family members and friends to also understand the nature of the problem. By having a better understanding of what their friend or relative is coping with, they will find themselves more able to help.

Is there a plan to the book?

Yes, there is, in as much as the book is divided up into sections. But please don't, for one moment, feel that this is one of those books that you have to read right through, from beginning to end. It quite definitely is not. It is a book for dipping into. If one particular subject – for example, the treatment of arthritis – interests you, just simply look for that section in the contents list and skip through until you find the question answered.

If I find, when reading the book, that a certain treatment that I'm receiving from my doctor appears to be at variance with what you are suggesting, what should I do?

Hopefully, this problem will not arise, since it has been my intention throughout the book to describe and encapsulate present medical thinking. However, if, for any reason, you are uncertain or confused by certain statements, continue to carry out the advice given to you by your doctor. Then, on your next visit to the surgery, bring up the point in question and ask his advice. Because, although I have tried to give the best advice, there is always the possibility – as in any book – that confusion may have occurred.

So I must finally emphasize that it is important, before you act upon any advice given in this book, that you consult your doctor.

What is Arthritis?

What is arthritis?

When trying to understand the meaning of medical words the first step is often to split the word into its component parts. Thus, the word 'arthritis' divides into, 'arthr-' and 'itis'. 'Arthr-' comes from the Greek *arthron*, meaning joint. There are over 200 joints in the body – some more readily recognizable than others. Essentially, a joint allows for the movement of one bone upon another. The knee joint is a good example of a typical joint, because it allows the lower leg to flex and extend upon the upper leg with complete stability. But there are many other, less obvious joints, such as those that allow the bones of our spinal column to move upon each other when we bend our backs.

In general terms, the suffix '-itis' refers to either an inflammation or infection, but in the context of the word 'arthritis' it has come to broadly represent the malfunctioning of a joint. So, I don't feel that the word 'arthritis' presents too much of a problem because it literally means what it says, the malfunction or disease of a joint. However, what I *would* like to do at this stage is to make quite sure that the distinction between two sorts of arthritis is fully under-stood, because it is absolutely crucial that their differences are appreciated before we go any further.

The reason for this distinction is because the treatment of these two forms of arthritis is often different.

You've probably come across both of them. They are osteo-arthritis and rheumatoid arthritis.

What is osteoarthritis?

Again, let's look at the roots of the word. The Latin word *os* means bone, and so 'osteoarthritis' would appear to mean inflammation of the joint and in the bones, surrounding the joint.

To a very limited extent, this is true. But there is one crucial element in the equation that has been omitted, and that is cartilage. Cartilage is a connective tissue that overlies the ends of some bones.

The reason why the normal knee joint does not grate is because these cartilage-capped bones can slide easily over each other. But – and this is the crucial element in osteoarthritis – if the cartilage becomes worn down and allows the hard ends of the bones to grate against each other the characteristic symptoms of pain and joint immobility result.

So, just to recapitulate, osteoarthritis arises in a joint whose cartilaginous surfaces have become eroded, leaving the bare ends of the bones to rub against each other.

It's worth noting that, in this variety of arthritis, there is certainly no infection and minimal inflammation.

What is rheumatoid arthritis?

I just mentioned that the ends of the bones that articulate, or 'glide' over each other, at the joint are capped with cartilage and that it is the free flow of these cartilaginous surfaces over each other that allows for easy movement of the joint.

This is true, but there is one further element to be taken into account – namely that in order to move freely a joint needs lubrication, in much the same way as the pistons in a car engine must have lubrication, in the form of oil in order to move easily within their respective cylinders.

Joints that have a wide range of movement, such as the knee joint, have their own lubricating fluid known as the synovial fluid. This fluid bathes the cartilaginous bone ends and is an elegant element in the smooth articulation of these joints. To prevent the fluid from leaking away, a capsule surrounds the joint, the inner lining of which is called the synovial membrane – a thin, transparent tissue that produces the synovial fluid.

In rheumatoid arthritis, it is the synovial membrane that becomes inflamed and which, in turn, causes the joint to malfunction.

What is rheumatism?

Many centuries ago, rheumatism was thought of as a flowing of unhealthy humours or vapours through the body. The word described non-specific symptoms of illness. So the word rheumatism has become synonymous with general aches and pains, though latterly it more specifically describes these symptoms in bones, joints, muscle and other soft tissues with no apparent under-lying illness.

What are the common symptoms of osteoarthritis?

As I have already explained, osteoarthritis is not an inflammatory process but rather a degenerative process – the cartilage actually wears down. Unlike rheumatoid arthritis, there are rarely any constitutional or systemic symptoms. Although there may be pain and immobility of the joint, this is not accompanied by general feelings of fatigue or perhaps even a temperature, loss of appetite, nausea, and feelings of being unwell and depressed.

With osteoarthritis, pain in a joint is the prominent feature. In the early stages of the disease, there may be no pain in the resting joint. Only movement of the joint will bring on the pain. As the disease progresses, however, there may be pain, even in the resting joint – this will be exacerbated by movement and relieved by resting the joint.

In osteoarthritis morning stiffness may be experienced. This is also a symptom of rheumatoid arthritis. But in osteoarthritis, the stiffness tends to wear off much more quickly and is certainly not so persistent.

Although osteoarthritis can occur as a symmetrical disease, unlike rheumatoid arthritis it tends to start off asymmetrically, involving the joints of just one particular part of the anatomy. A very common site for this to occur is in the hand, though here, interestingly, the distribution of affected joints will differ from rheumatoid arthritis. Your doctor will in fact sometimes be able to differentiate between the two diseases simply from the particular joints that are affected.

Other joints that can be typically affected in osteoarthritis are the hip joints, the knee joints, the ankle joints and the joints of the foot together with the shoulder joints, the elbow joints and the joints that allow the jaw to articulate with the skull.

Although the same joints can be involved in both rheumatoid arthritis and osteoarthritis, therefore, both the pattern in which they are involved and especially the asymmetrical way in which, in osteoarthritis, the joint involvement presents itself can readily differentiate between the two.

As I have mentioned earlier, osteoarthritis does not have any systemic features so that, unlike rheumatoid arthritis, there is no effect on the eyes, heart, lungs, or kidneys.

What are the common symptoms of rheumatoid arthritis?

It is important to realize that before any of the more obvious clinical features of rheumatoid arthritis appear, there may have been symptoms present for some time that the patient did not associate with rheumatoid arthritis. Sometimes it is only with hindsight that these can be seen to have been the start of the illness. Included among such symptoms are fatigue, weight loss, muscular aches and pains, and abnormal sweating, together with a general feeling of not being 'quite one's self'.

One very common symptom associated with rheumatoid arthritis is morning stiffness. Most of us, when we get up in the morning, will on occasion feel fairly stiff. This may be one of the reasons why we stretch, to relieve ourselves of this stiffness.

However, the morning stiffness associated with rheumatoid arthritis is not normally relieved by stretching. It is an exaggerated stiffness that tends to remain for three or more hours.

In association with this morning stiffness, one or more of the small joints of the hands or the feet are painful when moved and tender when touched. There may also be some swelling around these joints.

One of the most characteristic features of the way in which rheumatoid arthritis shows itself – and differs from osteoarthritis –

is that the joints are symmetrically affected. For example, if the joints of your left hand show symptoms of rheumatoid arthritis, the same joints of your right hand will also probably be affected.

Are there any other ways in which rheumatoid arthritis can show itself?

Yes, there are various other symptoms that can precede the onset of rheumatoid arthritis. These include pain in muscles, with or without a fever and sometimes with enlarged lymph glands. But I must emphasize that just because you have such symptoms does not mean to say that you are going to get rheumatoid arthritis. The symptoms that lead to such a diagnosis must be considered over a period of at least six to eight weeks, together with laboratory tests and X-rays, to give the complete clinical picture.

I mentioned earlier that one of the characteristic features of rheumatoid arthritis is that its appearance, in joints, is nearly always symmetrical. However, now and again, it can arise just in one joint – a problem that may present a diagnostic difficulty.

Rheumatoid arthritis may also, rarely, appear as carpal tunnel syndrome.

What is carpal tunnel syndrome?

The carpal tunnel is actually a little passageway through which some of the tendons to the hand pass. It also contains one of the main nerves that operates some of the muscles in the hand.

Any swelling within this confined space can result in compression of the nerve, together with a restriction of movement of the long muscle tendons – and this is carpal tunnel syndrome.

The compressed nerve in the carpal tunnel can produce numbness, tingling or pain in the hand and can also prevent some of the rather more delicate and intricate movements performed by a group of some of the small muscles of the hand. It is sometimes necessary for the fingers to receive passive exercises so that a full range of movements can be maintained.

Although carpal tunnel syndrome can be due to rheumatic disease there are other medical conditions that can give rise to it, including abnormal activity of the thyroid gland, pregnancy and injuries to the wrist. In most cases, however, the cause is never found. If you have been told that you have carpal tunnel syndrome, therefore, you must not immediately think, as many patients do, that you automatically have rheumatoid arthritis.

In most cases, the swelling within the carpal tunnel will go down of its own accord. Sometimes, however, when the problem becomes severe, and the structures within the carpal tunnel become very compressed, it may be necessary to consider surgery to relieve the pressure. The surgical operation is simple. A small incision is made into one of the ligaments surrounding the wrist joint, thereby relieving the swelling and pressure.

Can rheumatoid arthritis ever appear out of the blue?

Rarely. You might go to bed feeling relatively well, then, on awakening, find that you are so stiff that you can't get out of bed, and notice some pain and swelling in your joints. But more usually, the disease tends to creep up insidiously. In association with morning stiffness, you might simply find that one or more of the small joints of the hands or feet are painful when they are moved and feel tender when touched.

Once rheumatoid arthritis has started, how will it progress?

This is a very difficult question to answer because no two individual cases are the same and many factors may be involved. For example, the patient could also be suffering from another disease. Alternatively, certain treatments may not agree with the patient and may have to be stopped or there may be problems for the patient in actually receiving therapy. Also, some patients may not always keep to the prescribed treatment. All these, and many other external factors can, therefore, affect the natural progression of the disease, making the outcome of rheumatoid arthritis very difficult to predict. It is true to say, however, that in the majority of cases the disease can be contained and controlled with appropriate treatment.

There is an important point that must always be remembered when considering the progression of rheumatoid arthritis; namely that the disease tends to wax and wane. There are exacerbations and remissions and it is these remissions that sometimes make it difficult to be absolutely sure of the effectiveness of treatment, orthodox or otherwise, because there is sometimes no way of knowing whether or not remission would have been achieved without treatment or with an alternative therapy.

Apart from giving me joint problems, can rheumatoid arthritis affect other parts of my body?

Yes. It can cause several physical and psychological problems, including stress, anxiety and certain degrees of depression, all of which may be combined with a generalized feeling of fatigue. On top of this, because of the general debilitating aspects of arthritis, digestive problems may arise which can add to the general feeling of tiredness and fatigue. (For information on coping with depression, see p.109.)

Can arthritis affect my intelligence?

I can be quite categorical about this problem. Arthritis *never* directly affects a patient's mental capacity, though, of course, in some cases, due to psychological stress or generalized fatigue, the patient's mind might not be as alert as it normally is.

It is particularly important to emphasize the fact that somebody who is severely disabled by their arthritis – especially somebody who is confined to a life of virtual immobility – is in no way intellectually inferior. There seems to be a common assumption that people in wheelchairs, or who are otherwise physically deformed, are in some way mentally deficient. This is quite definitely not the case.

It is a message that has to be got over to employers, time and time again, that, just because somebody suffers from arthritis, it does not mean to say that their mental ability is any the less. Employers should never use arthritis as an excuse for criticizing an employee, especially on grounds of reduced intellectual capacity.

Is fatigue necessarily a part of having arthritis?

Yes. This is true for all types of arthritis, especially the more severe forms. In the early stages of arthritis this problem is often overlooked. Its importance, however, must be appreciated. For, unless there is a realization, early on, that fatigue is a part of the arthritic condition, it is all too easy to become depressed when once-easily completed tasks appear to be insurmountable.

Once fatigue is accepted as a definite part of arthritis, it becomes important to set aside certain periods of the day, and to give them over to adequate rest. Obviously, a lot will depend on the time you have available, but it is worth stressing that rest periods are an important part in the long-term treatment of arthritis. (For information on coping with fatigue, see pp.125.)

Can arthritis affect my eyes?

Yes. It is here, in fact, that one of the differences between rheumatoid arthritis and osteoarthritis lies, because it is rheumatoid arthritis rather than osteoarthritis, that affects the eyes. It is hardly surprising that this should be the case – the eye is made up of so many delicate structures that it invariably demonstrates some aspects of most diseases.

There are a number of ways in which rheumatoid arthritis can affect the eyes. Probably the most common problem is what is known as 'dry eyes' – a condition causing a sensation of grittiness in the eye on blinking, together with pain and irritation. This can have two causes: either not enough tears are being produced; or, if tears *are* being produced, they may not be adequately wetting the surface of the eye.

Normally, the tear glands are manufacturing tears which form a very thin tear film that is constantly passing over the front of the eye, acting as a comforting lubricant. If there is an insufficiency of this tear film, minute areas on the front of the eye become dry and it is these areas that transmit the sensation of grittiness.

Although the diagnosis of dry eyes is a fairly simple one to make, it is a good idea for all such patients to have at least one eye examination by an eye specialist to have the diagnosis confirmed and to ensure that there are no other underlying problems.

Is the eye examination painful?

No. The examination is a very simple one, normally involving the measurement of tear production by two small pieces of filter paper resting upon the inner lid of each eye for a minute or so.

Although there is no cure for dry eyes, the condition can be greatly helped by the frequent application of bland eye drops, in effect, tear substitutes. If frequent applications of these tear substitutes are inadequate there are further measures that can be taken, such as blocking the tear ducts to prevent those tears that are already formed from flowing away too easily.

In what other ways can rheumatoid arthritis affect my eyes?

Another way that rheumatoid arthritis can affect the eyes is by causing redness. Such redness must be taken very seriously and not simply put down to conjunctivitis. Although arthritic sufferers are just as likely as anybody else to get conjunctivitis but which require entirely different treatments.

One, known as iritis, is actually an inflammation within the eye. It is important that this condition be treated by an eye specialist for, if left untreated, complications can arise. The treatment itself is steroid drops together with drops that dilate the pupil but this may have to be continued for some weeks before the inflammation begins to subside.

The other two diseases that may be mistaken for conjunctivitis involve the white of the eye. It may seem strange at first sight, but this white of the eye, called the sclera, is, in fact, made up of the same sort of tissues as tendons and ligaments. As I have already described, rheumatoid arthritis, as well as being limited to certain joints, can also be a generalized disease. If it occurs in the eye it can give rise to inflammation on the white of the eye. In a mild and relatively harmless form this inflammation is called episcleritis while in its rather more severe form it is called scleritis. Both conditions should be assessed and treated by an eye specialist.

Can rheumatoid arthritis cause cataracts?

It is often assumed that cataracts and arthritis are related. This is not the case. It is, in the main, purely coincidental that these two quite distinct problems can occur in the same person. Some people also imagine that glaucoma and arthritis are in some way connected, but this again is a completely false assumption. However, cataracts can arise as a consequence of iritis and steroid treatment.

Which other sites in the body can be affected by rheumatoid arthritis?

The nerves may be involved. I have already explained one way in which this can happen – by the trapping of one of the major nerves to the hand, in carpal tunnel syndrome. There is also another way. The blood supply to the nerves may be slightly impaired, leaving areas of skin with decreased levels of sensitivity to various stimulae.

Another affected site is the lungs, where fluid may accumulate in a condition known as pleural effusion. Sometimes, too, fibrous tissue can be laid down in the lung tissue. A similar sort of fluid collection can occur around the heart and this is known as a pericardial effusion. On rare occasions, the kidney may be involved, and the patient is frequently found to be anaemic.

How does osteoarthritis differ from rheumatoid arthritis?

You will recall that I have said that to all intents and purposes osteo-arthritis is not an inflammatory process but, rather, a degenerative one. As such, unlike rheumatoid arthritis, there are rarely any general symptoms. In other words, although there may be pain and immobility of a joint, this is not accompanied by general feelings of fatigue, high temperature, loss of appetite, nausea, and feelings of being unwell or depressed. With osteoarthritis, pain in a joint is a prominent feature. Initially, in the early stages of the disease, there may be no pain in the resting joint – only movement of the joint brings on the pain. As the disease progresses, however, there may be pain, even in the resting joint, exacerbated by movement and relieved by resting the joint. When discussing rheumatoid arthritis, I mentioned the very typical morning stiffness associated with it. In osteoarthritis this morning stiffness may also be experienced, but it tends to wear off much more quickly than the morning stiffness of rheumatoid arthritis and is certainly not so persistent.

Another feature of osteoarthritis is that although it can occur as a symmetrical disease, unlike rheumatoid arthritis it tends to start off asymmetrically. A very common site for this to occur is in the hand. Interestingly, in the hand, the distribution of affected joints differs between rheumatoid arthritis and osteoarthritis, and your doctor may be able to differentiate between the two diseases from the particular joint distribution involved. Often, however, simple examination can not distinguish between the two conditions, in which case an X-ray of the hand will be necessary.

What joints can be affected in osteoarthritis?

Joints that can be typically involved are the hip joints, the knee joints, the ankle joints and the joints of the foot together with the elbow joints, the shoulder joints and the joints that allow jaw to articulate with the skull. So, although you can see that the same joints can be involved in both rheumatoid arthritis and osteoarthritis, both the pattern in which they are involved – and especially the asymmetrical way in which the joint involvement presents itself in osteoarthritis can differentiate between the two.

In passing, I should also emphasize that osteoarthritis does not have any systemic features so that, unlike rheumatoid arthritis, the eyes, the heart, the lungs and the kidneys are not normally affected.

General Clinical Aspects

What causes rheumatoid arthritis?

This is one of the major problems that still eludes us. Although much is known about the actual microscopical and biochemical progression of the changes that occur within the joint affected by rheumatoid disease, what exactly initiates the whole process is still not known.

It is clear that the answer to what causes rheumatoid arthritis is in some way connected with a phenomenon known as auto-immunity, and I think that it is important to explain what this means because it has wide medical ramifications.

Let us first consider what immunity entails. When a harmful bacterium enters the body the body protects itself by a process known as immunity. Immunity is performed by two separate systems working in harmony. There are the immunity cells – 'white cells' which circulate in the blood alongside the red blood cells – and the immunity antibodies – proteins, which also circulate in the blood.

When a harmful bacterium enters the body the antibodies neutralize it and prepare it for final elimination by the 'white' cells. Chemicals on the bacterium's outer wall, known as antigens, attract the antibodies, setting up what is called an antigen-antibody reaction. The 'white' cells are attracted to this area of antibody-antigen reaction and, as they begin to remove and eliminate the antibody-antigen complex, they initiate what is known as the inflammatory response.

But earlier I mentioned 'auto'-immunity. And this is the crucial point. Because, for some unknown reason, with this condition the immune system mistakes some of its own cells as foreign, as harmful, and sends off the antibodies and white cells to attack its own tissues. Currently, it is thought that it is this process that is at the basis of rheumatoid arthritis.

But this still does not answer the basic question of what actually starts this process of auto-immunity. In other words, what actually starts the body's defence mechanism turning upon its own tissues and cells. Current speculation surrounds the theory that an infecting organism such as a bacterium or a virus, when it settles upon the surface of the cells and tissues, can alter the chemical composition on the outside of the cells making up a particular tissue.

In the case of rheumatoid arthritis this would concern the cells of the synovial membrane of the joint. White cells and antibodies attack the altered synovial membrane, inciting an inflammatory response and so initiate the process that will eventually lead on to the full-blown clinical picture of the rheumatic joint.

However, this theory still leaves many important questions unanswered. For instance, it is well known in rheumatoid arthritis that the disease both waxes and wanes. So the question still remains, why does this inflammatory process seem to switch itself on and off? This is just one of the many basic questions surrounding the cause of rheumatoid arthritis to which there is still as yet, no known answer.

Is arthritis an inherited disease?

Heredity is always a difficult question because, in a number of diseases, inherited characteristics can skip one or more generations and can manifest themselves in dissimilar ways, in various generations. Sometimes members of a family can act as carriers of genetic faults and may themselves not be affected by the disease. There are also inherited characteristics that in themselves may be unconnected with a disease process but which may cause or precipitate an unconnected clinical problem.

An example of this is found with osteoarthritis. Certain families are without doubt prone to being overweight, which may or may not be totally a fault of the genes. Obesity can quite definitely exacerbate osteoarthritis of the hips and so, indirectly, a genetic link can be found between family members though not a directly inherited cause of the disease.

When searching for the cause of a disease geneticists can apply statistical analyses of familial studies as well as placing these familial studies within a particular social grouping or a particular environment. Not only can they seek genetic evidence of the occurrence of a disease from within a family but they can also elucidate what bearing genetics have upon that particular family's physical environment, dietary habits, occupational preferences, socio-economic status, their age and their sex, psycho-social factors and marital status. This overview is part of the science of epidemiology and when applied to the cause of rheumatoid arthritis it would appear that there is no evidence of it being a hereditary disease.

A rather sophisticated form of genetic studies involves looking at sets of twins, both identical (known as monozygotic twins), and non-identical (known as dyzygotic twins). When both sorts of twins are looked at, there does appear to be a slight increase in the incidence of rheumatoid arthritis in some twins. So what the geneticists have concluded is that there might be some element of genetic inheritance in such twins but not in the rheumatoid arthritic population as a whole.

There is one final point that I should like to make concerning the inheritance of rheumatoid arthritis. It has become evident that, in certain family groups, there is a predisposition towards the disease. But this predisposition is not the same thing as a direct genetic link.

Although it is true to say that rheumatoid arthritis is not an inherited disease one must, in fairness, make the proviso that due to a genetic predisposition, rheumatoid arthritis is more likely to occur in those families in which it has already occurred.

Can climate or physical environment have a bearing on one's rheumatoid condition?

For many years it was believed that rheumatoid arthritis was a disease of temperate climates and that by moving to warmer climates, nearer the equator, the arthritis would improve. But in recent years epidemiologists have quite clearly demonstrated that rheumatoid arthritis is no less common in warmer climates than in the colder climates. They have also shown that, in a slightly more specific way, urban and rural dwellers, whatever the kind of country they live in, are equally as likely to get rheumatoid arthritis.

There is no doubt, however, that cold and damp conditions do tend to exacerbate some arthritic conditions. But whether these climatic conditions are of primary or secondary importance, is impossible to say because we are all affected by weather to some extent. We all know that on a sunny summer's day we feel very much better than on a cold, wind-swept winter's day.

To a certain extent these feelings are psychological in nature. If spirits are already somewhat dampened by an acute exacerbation of arthritis it is reasonable to expect that having to endure it in conditions of damp and cold is hardly going to make the sufferer feel better. Whereas, on a hot sunny day, a general uplifting of spirits can often, temporarily, take the mind off the pain and disability of an arthritic condition.

In general terms, my advice is to try and keep as warm as possible, especially during the winter months. That does not just mean making sure that you are well wrapped up before going out, but also ensuring that in the home you try to avoid sitting in cold draughts and make the fullest possible use of whatever internal heating is available.

Can gout cause arthritis?

Yes, gout certainly can cause arthritis. In fact, it is actually a form of arthritis. As such, in its milder forms, gout can mimic osteo-arthritis. This is why it is important, if you feel that you have arthritis, not just to ignore it but to go to your doctor and make sure that your 'slight touch of arthritis', especially if it has suddenly appeared, is not gout. Although it may not be worrying you, it may be the first sign of gouty arthritis, a condition that can suddenly flare up overnight to leave you with an extremely tender joint.

Is the cause of gout known?

One of the things that differentiates gout from many of the other varieties of arthritis is that its cause can be definitely stated. In our circulating blood we have a low level of uric acid which is a byproduct of our body's nitrogen metobolism.

If there is a build-up of uric acid in the blood, due either to over-production or inadequate elimination, uric acid crystals, known as urates, tend to be deposited in the joints, and often into the joints of the big toe.

Underlying this problem of overproduction of urates or the problem of their elimination is normally a family history of gout. What probably happens is this. Patients, usually with a family history of gout and consequently with an elimination system that is unable to cope with high levels of uric acid, suddenly find themselves overwhelmed with a high level of uric acid in the blood. But this is not the whole story. There are many people with a predisposition to high uric acid levels who never develop gout. On the whole, then, gouty attacks arise from a predisposition to high levels of uric acid.

What are the other causes of gout?

These are many and varied, and include psychological and physical stresses. An example might be an operation, or the well-known excessive intake of food and alcohol. A doctor may also unwittingly precipitate an attack of gout by giving his patient a diuretic preparation (otherwise known as a 'water' tablet). This can cause gout by interfering with the kidney's ability to eliminate excessive amounts of urates. But the extraordinary thing is that, on the other hand, starvation or near starvation, as in somebody who is dieting, can also bring on an attack of gout.

Why is it that gout often occurs in the big toe?

Frankly, nobody knows, for sure. Why the big toe should be singled out is still a mystery, but when affected, it appears as an acutely painful and tender red swelling, the stretched skin above it being almost transparent. Often this can occur at night.

Although in certain cases gout can be confused with rheumatoid arthritis or even osteoarthritis, the classical manifestation of this problem normally leaves neither patient nor doctor in any doubt.

Can gout be easily treated?

Gout is now an eminently treatable disease, the more common drugs in use being allopurinol, colchicine and probenecid. An acute attack will normally necessitate complete rest of the affected joint (normally by slight elevation) combined with adequate doses of pain-killing and anti-inflammatory drugs. So, go and get those painful joints checked out, just in case you have got gout, because these treatments will give dramatic relief.

Is a painfully inflamed big toe always due to gout?

No. Other conditions can give rise to this clinical picture. It is very important when diagnosing the cause of this swollen joint to decide whether or not this is due to an infection, gout or arthritis. The problem may be septic arthritis. This is an acute emergency and must immediately be treated with antibiotics. Other possibilities are that the joint of the big toe has recently been injured or perhaps an old injury is now manifesting itself as osteoarthritis. There also is the possibility that the problem may be due to rheumatoid arthritis or it could even be due to pseudogout.

What is pseudogout?

With gout itself, the actual problem that makes the joint inflamed is the presence of urate crystals that set up the inflammatory reaction. In pseudogout – so called because of its similarity to gout – crystals of calcium pyrophosphate dihydrate precipitate out into the joint and, like the urate crystals of gout itself, set up an inflammatory reaction. Interestingly, the most common joint to be affected by pseudogout is the knee joint, the joint of the big toe being only rarely affected.

Unlike gout, for which there are specific drug treatments, pseudogout has to be treated symptomatically in that the joint must be rested when it is painful and pain-killing drugs given.

In particularly troublesome cases a needle may be inserted into the affected joint and fluid taken off. Local steroids may then be injected into the joint.

How may the arthritis of gout be differentiated from the other forms of arthritis?

One of the characteristic features of gout is that it appears suddenly – often at night and usually in one of the big toes in a patient who, up to that point, has not suffered from arthritis. Like osteoarthritis, it is normally an asymmetrical presentation, often occurring in only one joint.

The group of people in whom gout usually occurs, however, is different to that group in which rheumatoid arthritis occurs. Gout normally occurs in middle-aged and elderly men, whereas rheumatoid arthritis is found more commonly in women.

In addition, the arthritis that occurs in gout, even if untreated, normally only lasts for a matter of days or sometimes weeks, whereas the symptoms of rheumatoid arthritis tend to persist for a little longer than this.

Can arthritis cause back pain?

The best way to answer this question is probably in terms of two age groups: the younger and older.

In the younger age group it is important to appreciate that back pain is a relatively uncommon symptom, the spinal column of teenagers and people in their twenties and, to a certain extent, thirties, being a normal, physiologically non-rigid structure.

Although pain in this region may in a very few cases be the result of psychological problems such as depression or anxiety, it is normally symptomatic of specific back disease.

One such problem in younger people is known as spinal osteochrondritis and like so many others, its cause is unknown. The defect appears to lie in the parts of the vertebral bodies known as the epiphyseal end plates which are responsible for the growth of the vertebral bodies themselves. There is neither inflammation nor infection – rather, the laying down of the bone tissue seems to be disrupted and gives low back pain.

Another problem, in the younger age group is ankylosing spondylitis (see p.35).

What are other common causes of back pain in young people?

These tend to be either direct injury or prolonged chronic back strain that may result from, for instance, excessive weight training. At this stage, I should just like to mention two rare conditions over which there is sometimes some confusion: One is known as spondylosis and the other as spondylolysthesis. In spondylosis the articular joints between two vertebral bodies somehow become parted, separated. Following this instability, these vertebral bodies can slide apart, from each other, this being called spondylolysthesis. Slipped discs can also occur in this age group (see below).

What can cause back pain in older people?

Rheumatoid arthritis and osteoarthritis can cause back pain in older people, but there are other possible causes which I should like to discuss here.

One common cause of back pain is a slipped disc. I would like to start by describing what a slipped disc is, and then go on to mention the specific symptoms that can occur.

The vertebral spine is made up of a column of bones, sitting upon each other, and separating each bone is an intervertebral disc – in essence, a sort of shock absorber. What happens when you get a slipped disc is not that the actual disc slips away from its position between the two vertebral bodies but, rather, that the central part of the disc, known as the nucleus, protrudes or herniates out of a small weakness or defect in the outer coating of the disc.

When this occurs, back pain is experienced in the region of this defect. The pain can come on suddenly in association with a sudden or unwise movement of the back; it can appear without any apparent cause.

If slipped discs start in the back why can they cause pain in the leg?

The reason is this. The vertebral column contains the spinal cord. There are various gaps within the spinal column that allow the nerves of the spinal cord to travel out, from the column, between the vertebral bodies and off down the arms and legs to carry out various sensory and motor functions. When this disc material herniates out it can put pressure on one of these nerves as it passes out of its hole in the vertebral body. If a nerve is compressed in this way its functions will be impaired. While it will not totally lose all its actions, a relative mixture of its functions will certainly be lost. You might find, for example, that some of the muscles worked by the nerve lose their strength. This may cause a certain weakness in the particular leg that is affected. You may also find that the parts of the nerve that are responsible for conveying skin sensation from the leg are somewhat compromised and, as a consequence, you may notice areas of numbness over various parts of your leg.

In conclusion, then, a slipped disc will not only give you pain in the region of the lower back, but may also cause pain radiating to your buttocks or your lower leg. It may give your leg a certain weakness and numbness in areas.

What other causes are there of low back pain?

Perhaps the most obvious of all is disease of the bones themselves. Three diseases of bone that tend to occur in the older age groups are Paget's disease, osteomalacia and osteoporosis (see pp. 43, 44). All three can give low back pain.

There is one other problem that can occur with bone, however, and that is cancer. The cancers that arise in bone and give rise to low back pain are invariably secondary deposits from cancer elsewhere.

It is extremely unlikely if you have low back pain, however, that you have cancer.

Can back pain be due to causes other than the back itself?

Yes, low back pain can be nothing to do with the back at all, but can arise from other sites of the anatomy. Examples of this are pain from stomach ulcers, gynaecological disorders of the pelvis, the kidneys and pain arising from disease of the major arteries that traverse the abdomen.

What is ankylosing spondylitis?

Ankylosing spondylitis is a rheumatic condition that predominantly affects the axial skeleton. This means that the disease process is usually confined to the joints of the bones making up the spinal column, together with the joints connecting the spinal column to the pelvis, known as the sacro-iliac joints. The bones of the ribcage may also be involved.

Although the sacro-iliac joints allow for a certain amount of movement, they are much less flexible than the limb joints. Indeed, they are fairly inflexible.

When these diseased sacro-iliac joints are examined under the microscope, although, like rheumatoid arthritis, there is an inflammatory process taking place, it is most noticeable that there is an inflammatory process taking place, it is most noticeable that there is also an inflammatory process affecting the structures surrounding the outsides of these joints.

The structures affected are the ligaments that give strength and support to these joints as well as a membrane called the periosteum, which is an outer lining of tissue for the bones. Additionally, the cartilage within these joints is itself directly affected by the inflammatory process.

What subsequently tends to occur is that these inflamed tissues become less inflamed but laid down in their place is a fibrous tissue with much less elasticity than the tissues that it has replaced. This fibrous tissue, which is susceptible to calcium deposition, ends up in being ossified, which means that bone is actually formed within it.

So, what happens eventually, in the sacro-iliac joint, for instance, is that from being a joint with a certain amount of flexibility and elasticity, it becomes what is known as a fused joint. The joint is in effect, replaced by bone which gives rise to the variety of symptoms that I shall describe later.

What causes these specific joints to be affected in ankylosing spondylitis?

As with rheumatoid arthritis, the fundamental question as to what causes ankylosing spondylitis is unknown. But in the case of ankylosing spondylitis we have a clue that may eventually lead to the complete elucidation of the cause of this specific disease. For a specific chemical marker (known as the HLA B27 antigen) has been found on the surface of the cells in over 90 per cent of those who are diagnosed with the condition. I use the word 'marker' advisedly because it is not thought that the presence of this chemical on the surface of the cell membrane is a cause of the disease. But, it does at least take us one step further in trying to discover the basic cause of this problem.

If I have this chemical marker on the surface of my cells, how likely am I to contract ankylosing spondylitis?

Approximately 6 per cent of the population can be demonstrated to have this marker. But because you have this chemical marker on the surface of your cells does not mean that you are automatically going to get anklyosing spondylitis. Additional influencing factors are that the disease is more common in young men between the ages of 20 and 30 and that the condition shows a familial predisposition: families in which a member has ankylosing spondylitis show a greater preponderance of having similarly affected members.

What symptoms should I expect with ankylosing spondylitis?

The first signs of trouble tend to be an abnormal stiffening of the lower back together with pain, which, as the problem progresses, can also appear to be coming from the buttock area.

These symptoms can come on gradually but sometimes may appear suddenly in an acute form. The stiffness is normally worst in the morning.

Unlike many rheumatic diseases, the symptoms of anklyosing spondylitis are normally worse at rest and gradually improve with graduated exercises.

You mentioned that the ribcage may be involved in ankylosing spondylitis. Can this manifest itself in any way?

Yes, it can in that sometimes expansion of the chest in coughing, for example, may cause pain. This is due to inflammation of the small joints within the chest wall.

Can any other part of my body be affected?

Yes, the eyes can be affected. An inflammation can arise within the eye known as iritis (see p.23). This problem is usually signalled by redness of the eyes together with blurred vision and a dislike for bright light (known as photophobia).

Treatment involves the use of steroid drops and pupillary dilating drops. If you do have ankylosing spondylitis and have noticed that you have redness of the eyes it is mandatory that you seek specialist attention.

How may ankylosing spondylitis develop?

There are no clearly defined guidelines to this question, because the progression of the disease is very variable. In the majority of cases, although there may be remissions and relapses, the problem remains a mild one and may eventually resolve itself completely.

In a few cases, the joints of the spine may stiffen and the spine itself may become somewhat immobile. Such problems may often be overcome by the various treatment measures that I shall shortly discuss.

What treatment is available?

Like most treatments of rheumatic diseases, this problem falls into two parts: drug therapy and exercises.

First, drug therapy. With ankylosing spondylitis, anti-inflammatory drugs are given together with drugs for relieving the low back pain.

In addition to this specific drug therapy, is the all important advice about what can be done physically to ease the problem. The physiotherapist will give you a daily exercise programme that will allow you to maintain adequate mobility of the affected joints. One particular activity that is most helpful in this respect is swimming, since this allows for a fine balance between supporting the joints on the one hand, while promoting flexibility on the other.

Is there anything that I can do myself to help the problem?

Yes, there certainly is. Posture is all important. It is very important that you try consciously not to allow yourself to become stooped. So, when you are either standing or walking do try and maintain an erect posture. Although it may sound strange, posture is also important whilst you are sleeping. It is obviously impossible to actually correct your posture when you are asleep but you can do a great deal to improve matters by rearranging your sleeping circumstances: get a firm mattress and try using only one pillow. At all times while in bed, do try and prevent your back from becoming flexed and adopt the prone position as much as possible.

Should I worry unduly about my long-term prospects?

It is very important to remember, as stated above, that only a very few patients will suffer from anything but mild problems. For the majority of people with ankylosing spondylitis, as long as an adequate watching medical brief is kept upon the problem, it should not cause too much disability. Certainly most occupations can be carried out without too much alteration to the daily routine.

How likely are my children to get ankylosing spondylitis?

The chances of your child acquiring ankylosing spondylitis are probably less than one in ten, though if you are worried about this problem it is probably a good idea to undergo genetic counselling.

What are 'collagen' diseases?

The reason you may have come across so called 'collagen' diseases is that some of the diseases within this loose description can affect muscles and joints, giving aches and pains.

Some of the diseases grouped under this general heading are: systemic lupus erythematosus, systemic sclerosis, polymyositis, dermatomyositis, and polyarteritis nodosa. (These are also called connective tissue diseases.)

These diseases are rare and I shall not go into them in detail. I would, however, like to single out just one of them, systemic lupus erythematosus. This disease has recently become more widely recognized and, in its earlier stages, may be mistaken for rheumatoid arthritis. It is yet another example that emphasizes the advice I have given from time to time, in this book, about seeking medical advice rather than making a rough and ready diagnosis of one's own aches and pains as just being 'a touch of rheumatism'.

To return to systemic lupus erythematosus, you will recall that when I was talking about the cause of rheumatoid arthritis and mentioned the inflammatory process that takes place in rheumatoid joints, I stated that one of the possible causes for this inflammation was auto-immunity.

This would also appear to be the basis of the pathological process in systemic lupus erythematosus. In particular, what happens is that this auto-inflammatory process takes place in some of the smaller blood vessels, especially the smaller arteries. Thus there is inflammation in and around the arteries.

The manifestations of this disease are, in the main, the result of the interrupted blood supply to those areas of the body that are supplied by these inflamed and affected arteries.

Are there any particular people at risk from systemic lupus erythematosus?

Yes, There is a particularly vulnerable group – women between the ages of 20 and 40. A close look at statistics reveals that women within this age group are eight more times more likely to get systemic lupus erythematosus than men.

What symptoms may I expect from systemic lupus erythematosus?

With blood vessels supplying blood to every part of the body, it is theoretically possible for any organ or groups of organs to be affected. When systemic lupus erythematosus was first recognized as a disease, it was this 'multisystem' problem that was the predominant feature. It has now become recognized that systemic lupus erythematosus can exist as a mild disease and may not progress.

Early symptoms may be pains in the joints. These symptoms can be confused with those of rheumatoid arthritis or osteoarthritis. But your doctor will be aware of this fact and will know that, especially if you are a woman between the ages of 20 and 40, a diagnosis of rheumatoid arthritis should not be made until systemic lupus erythematosus has been excluded.

Another common way in which systemic lupus erythematosus may show itself is with an unusual skin rash, sometimes accompanied by hair loss. At the same time you might notice that you have a temperature that comes and goes. Sometimes, when your lymph nodes are up, which can also occur with this disease, you can be diagnosed initially as having a mild viral infection. So it is important, if these sorts of symptoms continue, that you consult your doctor.

Other symptoms include pain coming from the muscles, loss of appetite, even nausea and vomiting. Again, it is easy to confuse these symptoms with a typical viral illness, so consult your doctor if they persist. Although other parts of your body may be affected, such as your kidneys and your lungs, I don't propose to go into these symptoms in detail here. If such problems exist, your doctor wil undoubtedly go into more specific detail as to what is involved as regards symptoms and treatment.

Can pain arise from the bones themselves?

Yes. There are many diseases of the bones from which pain can arise. I shall mention three such diseases here. Two have similar names and are often confused: osteomalacia and osteoporosis.

The third disease is known as Paget's disease of bone.

However, before we go on, I should just like to describe the exact nature of bone. At first sight, it would appear to be an inert structure, a structure without life, but this is far from being the case. At any one time, bone cells known as osteoblasts and osteoclasts are continually remodelling the bone, laying down calcium from one part of the bone and taking it up from another. In every sense of the word, therefore, bone is a living tissue. A tissue that is made up of what is known as an osteoid matrix which is then calcified, or has calcium laid down in it. (It is this that gives bone its final strong characteristics).

In addition to this, in the centre of many long bones there is what is commonly called bone marrow. It is from this bone marrow that many blood cells are initially produced, together with many of the cells that are concerned in the body's defences.

With osteomalacia, the osteoid matrix itself is normal, but the process whereby the osteoblasts lay down the calcium salts is in some way defective. This results in the bones lacking strength. Surprisingly, this inability of the osteoid matrix to be calcified is not due to a lack of calcium but, rather, to a lack of vitimin D, an essential chemical in the calcifying process. It is this lack of vitamin D in children that is the cause of osteomalacia, which is otherwise known as rickets.

What can cause this lack of vitamin D?

It can be due to inadequate dietary intake. However, even though enough vitamin D is ingested, it is possible that due to an inability of the gastro-intestinal tract to absorb the vitamin D, not enough of it actually gets into the body. Sometimes, this lack of vitamin D can be due to kidney disease.

So, without this bony skeleton support, bone pain in osteo-malacia is a prominent symptom. The pain is characteristically found in the back, the hips, the ribs and the legs. In addition to these problems there is sometimes muscle weakness.

characteristically found in the back, the hips, the ribs and the legs. In addition to these problems there is sometimes muscle weakness.

How, then, can osteomalacia be treated?

As I have already stated, the primary cause of osteomalacia is, in most cases, lack of vitamin D. Once suitable doses of the vitamin have been administered, calcification of the osteoid matrix takes place.

What is osteoporosis?

As mentioned earlier, bone is essentially made up of the osteoid matrix, into which the calcium salts are deposited by the bone cells to give it strength. What occurs in osteoporosis is a partial loss of both the calcium salts and some of the osteoid matrix.

What causes osteoporosis?

Bones can lose some of their calcium and some of their osteoid matrix if there is not enough calcium in the diet or if the calcium is not absorbed into the body via the gastro-intestinal tract.

Osteoporosis can sometimes occur in cases where there has been prolonged immobility which, in certain clinical situations, can give rise to a vicious circle. For instance, if a patient is admitted to hospital with a fracture of the femur, which may well be in part due to osteoporosis, a prolonged stay in hospital together with the inherent immobility, can give rise to further osteoporosis. For this reason it is important to recognize and treat this condition.

It can also occur in certain post-menopausal women who have disease of their parathyroid glands (these glands have nothing to do with the thyroid gland although they are imbedded in the back of it).

Patients taking steroids are also at risk. As a consequence, patients with rheumatoid arthritis who take steroids may be placing themselves at risk of developing osteoporosis.

What symptoms does osteoporosis cause?

Commonly, the problem announces itself with backache, but fractures at the hip and the wrist can also occur.

How can the condition be treated?

Calcium, together with vitamin D, are given and it has been recently shown that oestrogens can help. Other measures such as ensuring that there is adequate mobilization are also of great importance.

What is Paget's disease of bone?

In Paget's disease the delicate balance of remoulding and reshaping of the bones is thrown into confusion, resulting in gross irregularities and deformities, and enlargement of the bones. The disease is more common in men, especially in older men, and it predominantly affects the bones of the spine, the skull and the bones of the legs.

What sort of symptoms can arise from Paget's disease?

Pain can arise from the deformities of the bones. This can be dull, aching and constant, especially from the back and in the legs.

One well known feature of Paget's disease is an increase in the size of the bones of the skull. In the old days, when men used to frequently wear hats, a well known pointer to Paget's disease was the information that the patient had found, of late, that he needed an increase in the size of his hat.

How may Paget's disease be treated?

It is now apparent that a hormone called calcitonin is of great value in treating this disease. Such treatment has to be closely monitored and is very much a matter of liason between your doctor and specialists in this field known as endocrinologists.

What about polymyalgia rheumatica and temporal arteritis?

The reason that these two diseases are often mentioned in the same breath is the fact that patients who are diagnosed as having polymyalgia rheumatica sometimes go on to acquire temporal arteritis, a disease that can have severe consequences.

Not only is it important to diagnose polymyalgia rheumatica, therefore, but it is equally important to bear in mind that this may lead on to temporal arteritis.

What is polymyalgia rheumatica?

As the name suggests, this is a problem that normally occurs as stiffness and pain in muscles, the groups of muscles most commonly affected being those of the shoulders, the neck, the back and the hips. What actually causes the problem is unknown for examination of the affected muscles under the microscope invariably shows little, if any, evidence of inflammation.

Does polymyalgia rheumatica come on quickly or slowly?

Either is possible. Normally, the history is one of a slow onset with often the muscles of one shoulder demonstrating pain and stiffness and then, some weeks later, the muscles of the other shoulder showing similar symptoms. Then, gradually, the neck, the back muscles and the muscles of the hip all follow suit.

This is why I must emphasize once again that it is terribly important not just to put such symptoms down to vague terms such as fibrositis until your doctor has given you a full examination.

Are there any other symptoms of polymyalgia rheumatica?

Yes. You may generally feel unwell, even depressed. You may also lose your appetite and experience some weight loss.

What is temporal arteritis?

Temporal arteritis can either come out of the blue of its own accord or follow on from polymyalgia rheumatica. Usually, it occurs as a headache. But unlike so many headaches, it tends to impart a certain exquisite tenderness to the skin over the temples so that activities such as putting on a hat or combing the hair become painful affairs.

How may these two diseases be treated?

Both polymyalgia rheumatica and temporal arteritis are treated with steroids such as prednisolone tablets. Although steroids can have side-effects, their dosages are kept to a minimum to avoid such problems.

What is fibrositis and how can it be treated?

Fibrositis is one of those medical words with no real scientific basis that has, over the years, developed a popular meaning. Originally it was believed that there was a condition with this name, caused by inflammation in the fibrous tissues and, although there is now no evidence to support this, the term is still retained.

In general, however, fibrositis refers to rheumatological pain that does not arise as a part of arthritic disease, although, of course, there may be a joint problem present.

To most people it describes a generalized pain, usually sited in the shoulders and neck, the upper arms, the chest muscles and in the lower back. One very characteristic feature that I have noted, over the years, is that the pain is often described as 'always' being there – a nagging pain, which, in some cases, can be a constant worry. Other problems involve sleep disturbance and, in some cases, I have known the persistence of the symptoms to lead to depression.

I think that probably the most annoying feature of fibrositis is the fact that it usually has no apparent specific cause. All the usual tests seem to be normal – an extraordinary fact, considering the nature of the problem and the large numbers of people who suffer from the condition.

There is an important fact that must not be lost sight of; namely, that is a mistake to label a patient's symptoms as fibrositis until one can be quite certain that there is no other, underlying problem. Equally, it is important that people with the symptoms of fibrositis do not just label themselves with this tag and decide not to bother their doctor, because similar symptoms may herald a specific disease such as polymyalgia rheumatica (see p.45) which will require further medical assessment.

But what of the treatment of this condition? As with so many medical conditions, where the cause is ill-defined or frankly unknown, treatment presents a problem. It is, inevitably, difficult to treat an unspecified illness, a fact that may allow the unscrupulous to suggest or advise any number of unproven treatments.

A further factor in the equation is that people with fibrositis are often dubbed as having a psychological problem, which is quite definitely not the case, although it *is* true to say that a depressive illness may arise because of the fibrositis.

Because of the rather obscure nature of fibrositis successful treatment is frustrating to both patient and doctor alike. Some patients respond well to treatment such as ultrasound and microwave therapy as well as the more traditional remedies of superficial thermal applications, linaments and massage.

Is frozen shoulder due to arthritis?

Frozen shoulder is not due to arthritis, in the sense that the articular surfaces of the bones of the shoulder joint show the changes normally seen in arthritis. It is understandable that confusion arises because the symptoms of frozen shoulder – a certain immobility of movement of the shoulder girdle together with pain, to varying degrees – are very similar to the symptoms found in an arthritic joint.

The symptoms of frozen shoulder come from the soft tissues surrounding the shoulder joint, known as the capsular tissues. Local tissue injury or inflammation tend to cause problems in the capsular tissue but in extreme cases fracture of the humeral bone, cervical disc disease or even a stroke can be rare causes of frozen shoulder.

Treatment of the problem is a two-pronged affair. Firstly, the joint is eased into action by the use of steroids (see p.66), injected directly into the capsular tissue. Secondly, the rehabilitative programme is completed by mobility-producing exercises. Recovery may take some time but, as many of the patients are in the younger age groups, full movement nearly always returns.

Are corns due to arthritis or can they herald arthritis?

Although arthritic sufferers appear to be more prone to corns, corns are definitely not due to arthritis.

A corn is an area of hardened skin. It is one of Nature's protective mechanisms and ensures that an area of skin which it subject to pressure and subsequent damage is hardened, to protect both itself and its underlying structures.

Is there a connection between rheumatoid arthritis and rheumatic fever?

This is an example of similar words being used in medicine to describe two completely dissimilar conditions for there is no connection between rheumatoid arthritis and rheumatic fever. However that is not to say that, in a few patients, the two diseases may not be present.

Rheumatic fever normally occurs in children. It is caused by streptococcal bacteria which, as a consequence of their toxic effects, can cause damage to both the heart and the kidneys, resulting in cardiac and renal disease.

Is there any connection between the menopause and arthritis?

Yes, there certainly is. This is especially the case in osteoarthritis, where the hormonal changes in the body during the menopause appear to bring about definite change in the cartilage tipped bones, within the joints – especially the fingers, thumbs, knees and neck.

The menopause tends to have very little effect on rheumatoid arthritis.

Does swelling of the legs and ankles always indicate arthritis?

Swelling of the limbs and ankles can indeed be due to rheumatoid arthritis or osteoarthritis. If you experience these symptoms, it is important that you consult your doctor even if you have already had arthritis diagnosed, because swelling of the legs and ankles can also be an initial symptom of conditions such as heart disease, liver disease or kidney disease.

Before going any further, it is important to mention that by far and away the most common cause of swelling of the legs, and especially the ankles, is faulty posture. As we all get older, the mechanism whereby the body pumps excessive fluid from our limbs back up to our heart can sometimes begin to fail, as can the valves in the veins, in the legs, which are an integral part of this system.

If you do have persistent swelling in your legs and ankles, especially if it appears to be painless and persistent, then it is important that you let your doctor know so that he can pinpoint the cause.

Do lumps in the skin, especially near joints, mean that I have arthritis?

Hard nodules are sometimes found just beneath the skin in certain forms of arthritis, including arthritis caused by gout. These nodules tend to appear after the arthritis has been present for some little time and, by the time that they arise, there is usually no doubt about the diagnosis.

The common lumps that you may find around your joints, especially in the hand, are called ganglia. They are of no consequence and do not mean that you are liable to get arthritis.

Are pains in the skin always due to arthritis?

No, not always. Here, we are talking about something very specific. Not the deep-seated pain that is associated with arthritis, but superficial pain – pain in the skin itself. If such symptoms are experienced it is probable that the cause is some sort of malfunction of the nerves running in or just beneath the skin.

A common example of this is shingles, especially the shingles that affects the chest and abdomen.

Before the skin manifestations of shingles become apparent, there is often a prolonged period of pain which is often put down to some sort of rheumatic condition, even by the doctor who has examined his patient carefully. Once the manifestations of shingles become apparent, the cause of the problem is realized.

If you experience an unusual, superficial pain, that appears to be situated just in or beneath your skin, and it persists, consult your doctor, and don't simply put it down to fibrositis or rheumatism.

Are tennis elbow and golfer's elbow forms of arthritis? Are they likely to lead to arthritis in later life?

One of the most important things to remember about joint pain is that the pain can come from both the joint itself and the tissues surrounding the joint. Tennis elbow and golfer's elbow are both good examples of soft tissue injury around the joint, and so are not due to arthritis of the joint. Like frozen shoulder, tennis and golfer's elbow can often be greatly helped by local injections of cortisone and the chances of developing arthritis in the joint is slight.

What is bursitis?

This is a good example of a word thrown at you by the medical profession when you have gone along to your doctor thinking that you have some form of arthritis because, say, you have swelling around your knee joint. He might even enlarge upon the diagnosis by telling you that you have got housemaid's knee. It's quite reasonable to assume that the whole thing is connected with arthritis. But it is not. People with bursitis are no more likely to have arthritis than anybody else. In fact, a bursa is a little fluid-filled sac, collections of which tend to congregate in areas where muscular tendons are prone to chafing.

All that happens when you get bursitis is simply a slight swelling of one or more of these sacs, which normally settles in its own good time as long as the affected part of the body is given adequate rest.

Do pins and needles in my limbs indicate that I have arthritis?

In certain circumstances such sensations can accompany arthritis. One very specific form of osteoarthritis, which affects the thumbs, gives a definite pricking sensation at or near the base of the thumb. This may necessitate further supportive treatment in the form of a thumb splint.

As for pins and needles generally, these are not normally an indication of arthritis as such, although they can be experienced in the earlier stages of rheumatoid arthritis. Pins and needles are far more likely to be a manifestation of pressure on a nerve and, if only intermittent and slight, are not to be taken too seriously. If they persist, however, and are associated with other areas of similar sensations in other parts of your body, these symptoms should be reported to your doctor.

Are the cracks that I hear coming from my joints from time to time anything to do with arthritis? If I have them am I more likely to get arthritis?

Certainly people with arthritis, and especially those with osteoarthritis, are prone to these noises that can come from any joint at any time. In the majority of people – certainly in the majority of the elderly such creaks and cracks become increasingly common and, in most cases, there is no association between these noises and any major form of arthritis. They are far more likely to be a sign of old age just simply creaking on. Such joint noises can occur in any age group, however, and should not be taken too seriously.

If someone is double-jointed, does it mean that they are more prone to arthritis in later life?

There is little evidence to suggest that people who are double-jointed will, in later life, develop arthritis, though it is probably a good idea to dissuade those children who delight in demonstrating their ability to bend their fingers at extraordinary angles not to do so. Such abnormal positions are probably not, in the long run, particularly helpful in the child's development.

My children had growing pains. Does this mean they are more prone to getting arthritis in later life?

It is now becoming evident that growing pains are a normal phenomenon in growing children. It is not unusual for a child, at some time or another, to complain that he or she has vague aches, more often than not in the arms and the legs. There is no evidence, at present, to suspect that such children will, in later life, go on to develop either rheumatoid arthritis or osteo-arthritis. Neither is there any evidence to suggest that if you or a family member suffers from arthritis, your child stands a greater risk of developing the problem.

There is a small group of children, however, in whom growing pains do in fact turn out to be the first symptoms of juvenile arthritis. It is as well, therefore, even if the growing pains do not seem to be concerning the child, to take the child to your doctor, for reassurance more than anything else.

Are the cramps that I get in my legs at night anything to do with my arthritis?

Leg cramps can be one of a number of causes of lower limb pain. Under these circumstances, it is important that you tell your doctor of the problem for, in most cases, leg cramps can quite easily be relieved by taking quinine tablets, before you retire, at night.

As to whether leg cramps have any specific association with arthritis, and, in particular, rheumatoid arthritis, this is a matter for debate.

It is often difficult to pinpoint the cause of this supposedly simple condition. Leg cramp can arise in the legs of someone who has no rheumatic disease. But in conjunction with rheumatoid arthritis, with the stiffening of joints, muscular spasms may follow, and it is then difficult to decide whether such symptoms are due to rheumatoid disease or the so-called 'normal' nightly leg cramps.

This is often a difficult problem to unravel but in most cases there is certainly no harm in the patient with rheumatoid arthritis trying a course of quinine tablets to see whether or not the symptoms are relieved.

If I have arthritis is this the only cause of pains in my legs?

One of the problems and, indeed, one of the major pitfalls, of medical diagnosis, is to fall into the trap of assuming that once you think that you have discovered a cause for a patient's symptoms you have solved the problem itself.

It is quite possible, for instance, that osteoarthritis of the knee joint has been correctly diagnosed, but that the possibility has been overlooked of a second and quite unconnected cause for your symptoms which mimic the symptoms of your osteoarthritis.

A good example of such a disease is a vascular condition known as claudication of the leg, where the blood vessels in the leg can become partially blocked. Without a proper supply of oxygen pain is felt in the leg, more often than not, when walking.

If you are getting pains in your leg and you have decided that they are rheumatic in origin, it is, therefore, possible that you are mis-diagnosing yourself.

You may be overlooking the possibility of vascular disease, as I have just described.

On the other hand, if you have been to your doctor, and he has made a diagnosis of osteoarthritis, but you find that the treatment that he has given you does not seem to be helping the problem, it is important that you go back to him, and explain that the symptoms have not subsided. On this second consultation, even if he did not do so on the first occasion, he will undoubtedly check the pulses in your legs, to make sure that you have adequate blood flow.

There are all sorts of other causes of pains in the legs – which, if not seen to, can lead on to serious consequences.

There are several possibilities. You might have thrombosis of the veins – either the superficial veins or the deeper veins within the substance of the leg – or you could have a trapped nerve in your lumbar spine, the pain of which can manifest itself as pain in the leg. It is equally possible that you may just be getting night cramps, or that the pain may be the first warning of an impending ulcer. Or the whole problem may quite simply be due to bulging varicose veins.

If you do have pains in your lower limbs, therefore, don't just put it down to some vague rheumatism or rheumatic problem. Go and see your doctor. If, having seen him, the pain persists, go back for further advice for your doctor will know what sort of problems can arise in your lower limbs and, if the treatment is not working, will wish to examine you once more.

Can children get arthritis?

Yes, a form of arthritis does occur in childhood. It was formerly called juvenile rheumatoid arthritis but is also known as juvenile chronic arthritis. It is not exactly similar to rheumatoid arthritis of adulthood.

What, then, are the differences between rheumatoid arthritis found in the adult and the child?

You will recall that I mentioned that there are two major components that make up rheumatoid arthritis in adulthood:

on the one hand, the specific problems that relate to the joints and, on the other, the general symptoms that affect the whole body, such as fatigue and anaemia as well as specific organs including the lungs, heart and kidneys. (These general effects are also often described as systemic effects.)

In the majority of cases of adult rheumatoid arthritis, the effects are predominantly in the joints. Some patients will have no systemic effects at all while others will have a variety of symptoms ranging from the very mild to the severe.

In juvenile rheumatoid arthritis, it is the systemic effects that can be more noticeable than the joint problems. In fact, sometimes the systemic manifestations are the first to appear and it may be these which first alert the doctor to the possibility of juvenile rheumatoid arthritis. For instance, a fever without any other symptoms can appear, sometimes rising to quite high temperatures, before the true nature of the disease is appreciated. As a consequence, the problem can easily be put down to either a bad cold or influenza.

A further problem can arise in the presence of a high fever together with a tender joint, for a doctor can make the mistake of diagnosing joint infection. To complicate matters even further, a rash can occur over the skin of a child, with or without a temperature, in association with enlarged lymph glands, all of which may lead to the diagnosis of an infection rather than the hidden diagnosis of juvenile rheumatoid arthritis.

Can juvenile rheumatoid arthritis affect children's eyes?

Yes, it can. Once again, the way in which juvenile rheumatoid arthritis manifests itself here, differs from the problems of adulthood.

Some children are found to have an inflammation within their eyes, known as iritis. This, when examined microscopically, is, in general terms, the same sort of process that takes place in the inflamed arthritic joints. In children it occurs in its chronic rather than acute form though this makes it no less potentially hazardous. As a consequence, it is important that every child with rheumatoid arthritis is seen by an eye specialist for signs of eye inflammation.

If a child has juvenile rheumatoid arthritis does this mean that he will be crippled for life?

One of the important things to realize, right from the start, about juvenile rheumatoid arthritis is the prognosis, or forecast of the outcome of the disease.

In juvenile rheumatoid arthritis, the prognosis, in the majority of cases, is good. Most of the children will go into remission having, for a variable time, been treated for the disease. Official figures show that 70-75 per cent of all children who are diagnosed as having juvenile rheumatoid arthritis recover completely from this disease. Therefore, much of what I have said and am going to say will apply only to that small minority in whom the problem persists.

Are there different forms of joint problem in juvenile rheumatoid arthritis?

In certain respects, yes. One of the features that differentiates juvenile rheumatoid arthritis from the adult variety is that, in the juvenile form, it is more common for four or less joints to be initially affected. The problem often arises in just one joint, this normally being the knee joint, whereas in adult rheumatoid arthritis it is not uncommon to find many more than four joints simultaneously affected.

At this stage, I shall not go into the various laboratory tests that have been carried out. But one interesting fact is that the majority of adult patients with joint inflammation are found to have a rheumatoid factor in their blood while only a minority of those with juvenile rheumatoid arthritis have similar results.

So really, from what you have said, the outlook for a child with juvenile rheumatoid arthritis is not hopeless?

Far from it. With modern treatment and active physiotherapy most, if not all, of the problems can be overcome.

Therapy

What happens if I am diagnosed with rheumatoid arthritis?

When you go to your doctor and the diagnosis of rheumatoid arthritis is made, perhaps after some weeks and following a number of blood tests together with a series of X-rays, you might well be started on a course of aspirin.

But why, following all these highly scientific tests, will my doctor put me on a course of simple aspirin? Surely modern medicine has more to offer me than this?

At first sight, when we see the marvels of medical science, it might seem strange to begin with simple aspirin. But this drug has an important place in the treatment of arthritis for it is not just, as many people suppose, a pain-killer. It is also a drug that can directly reduce the inflammatory response, especially of joints with rheumatoid arthritis.

It is true that aspirin has been around for a long time. In its crudest form – an extract from the bark of the willow tree – it has been available since the times of the ancient Greeks. Its use became widespread in the eighteenth century and in Germany, in the mid-nineteenth-century, it was chemically refined as salicylic acid. It has been used in this form, ever since, as both a pain-killer and as an anti-inflammatory drug.

But just because aspirin has been around for a long time does not mean to say that it is old-fashioned or obsolete. On the contrary, it has handsomely stood the test of time. We still do not really know how it works, but it appears to somehow inhibit chemicals around the inflamed joints, called prostaglandins, that are thought to be the initiators of the inflammatory process.

Does aspirin have any side-effects?

Like most drugs with a worthwhile and sustained effect, aspirin does have side-effects. Perhaps the most annoying of these are the symptoms of indigestion or dyspepsia. These are caused by irritation of the stomach lining, which may seem, at first sight, somewhat contradictory, as aspirin is an anti-inflammatory drug.

As well as this problem, aspirin can cause bleeding from the tiny blood vessels just beneath the lining of the stomach wall. In most cases this is so mild that it goes unnoticed, but sometimes, one of the larger blood vessels of the stomach wall can be eroded, causing considerable loss of blood which passes into the intestine. Because this fresh blood has to travel completely through the intestinal tract, by the time it is passed out (in the faeces), it gives the stools a black colour. So, if you are taking aspirin and notice that you are passing black faeces, alert your doctor at once. Considerable amounts of blood can be lost 'silently' in this way, and can leave a patient severely anaemic, which, in itself can be a serious problem – particularly since patients with rheumatoid arthritis tend to be slightly anaemic anyway. This on top of blood loss from the gastro-intestinal tract can have serious and far-reaching effects.

What other side-effects can I expect from aspirin?

One of the more common side-effects experienced by patients taking aspirin to reduce the pain and inflammation of their rheumatoid arthritis is a sensation of ringing in the ears, called tinnitus. The reason why most people do not get tinnitus when they take aspirin for headaches and other minor aches and pains is because they are not taking it at the higher dosage levels normally used for rheumatoid arthritis.

Hearing may also be affected but, both this and the sensation of ringing in the ears, does not indicate any permanent damage to the hearing apparatus. Hearing will return to normal and the tinnitus disappear with either cessation of the aspirin or a reduction in the drug's dosage.

Other, much rarer, side-effects of aspirin include an allergic response, and in very rare cases both the liver and the kidneys can be damaged. It should always be remembered, however, that almost any drug that enters the body's bloodstream can interact with other drugs being taken at the same time. As far as aspirin is concerned, although it can react with many drugs, the two groups of drugs that your doctor will closely monitor are those concerned with controlling diabetes mellitus and those concerned with preventing abnormalities in the blood's clotting mechanism.

Can aspirin have any beneficial side-effects?

At the present time there are a number of clinical trials taking place to establish whether aspirin, in smaller doses than those taken for the control of rheumatoid arthritis, can prevent coronary thrombosis and strokes. It is believed that aspirin reduces the adhesiveness of certain blood-clotting cells called platelets and, as a consequence, reduces the formation of the small cellular clots that are the ultimate cause of so many heart attacks and strokes.

Is there any way in which aspirin can be chemically modified to eliminate some of these side-effects?

Yes. Several ingenious methods have been tried, some more successfully than others. For example, various coatings have been used in attempts to prevent gastric irritation as well as chemically manipulating the drug to best effect in the acid environment of the stomach and the alkaline environment of the intestine. Paracetamol is an alternative oral therapy. It is said not to have anti-inflammatory activity; only pain-killing effects. Many physicians will prescribe paracetamol as a drug of first choice in patients with mild rheumatoid arthritis for it does seem to have a limited anti-inflammatory action as well as having the great advantage of not causing dyspepsia, to any great degree. However, paracetamol can have severe effects on the liver, especially in cases where there is already some liver damage, and although the drug would appear to be innocuous, being obtainable without a doctor's prescription, its liver toxicity must always be borne in mind.

How is the child with juvenile rheumatoid arthritis treated?

Many of the same drugs and the techniques of physiotherapy that are used to treat adult rheumatoid arthritis are utilized in this younger group of patients.

Aspirin has an important role to play in the treatment of juvenile rheumatoid arthritis. Recently, there have been reports that aspirin can cause an illness in children known as Reye's Syndrome. There has been no conclusive evidence in this country that large doses of aspirin given to children with juvenile rheumatoid arthritis can induce this illness, but an association between taking aspirin and Reye's Syndrome has been highlighted.

The question is still debatable and you and your children must be guided by your consultant on whether or not it is advisable to take aspirin on an individual basis.

Are there any other tablets that can reduce the pain and inflammation of rheumatoid arthritis?

You may have come across the term 'non-steroidal anti-inflammatory drugs' (often referred to as NSAIDs). This is quite a mouthful, but it is a useful classification of some of the drugs that can be used in rheumatoid arthritis.

If you have been treated for rheumatoid arthritis for any length of time, you will undoubtedly have been treated with either one or more of these drugs. There are a great many of them – ample testimony to the fact that there is no single, simple miracle drug. Indeed, one of these NSAIDs, called phenylbutazone – originally hailed as a wonder drug – has recently been withdrawn because of its harmful side-effects.

All this demonstrates the importance of each patient being assessed, on an individual basis, by their doctor rather than receiving a cocktail of tablets because their doctor feels that such drug combinations 'normally do the trick in the majority of patients'.

However, the choice of which drug to use is often made on less than medical grounds. The doctor may only have a limited experience with some of these drugs and be unwilling to subject his patients to newer preparations. In some cases, he may be quite right, but in the process he could well be overlooking a newer drug which might in the long run, become an established and beneficial treatment for rheumatoid arthritis. If you hear of a new drug for rheumatoid arthritis, therefore, write down its name and the next time you visit your doctor ask his opinion about it.

Another consideration affecting the choice of drug may be expense. This should not enter into any treatment for any disease but it invariably does. Drug companies are often (in my opinion, unfairly) blamed for profiteering but in many cases the development of a drug costs them many millions of pounds, and they obviously have to recoup their capital outlay. Hence the high costs of some drugs which are unobtainable from the National Health and which, in my opinion, should be readily available if proved to be of benefit to patients, however expensive.

Why is phenylbutazone no longer available?

Its side-effects were considered too dangerous to allow its general use. The minor side-effects of phenylbutazone are a tendency to cause dyspepsia and fluid retention, which, in the elderly, can contribute to heart failure. But by far and away its most serious side-effect is that in a small proportion of patients it causes the complete suppression of production of the body's blood cells. The cells are produced in the bone marrow and without them no red cells or white cells can be produced and enter into the bloodstream. This condition is known as aplastic anaemia and although it can be treated by a bone marrow transplant as a form of therapy this is not always successful.

However, there are other NSAIDs with similar anti-rheumatic properties to phenylbutazone which can adequately take its place.

Is there any one particular drug that is representative of the 'non-steroidal anti-inflammatory' drugs?

Personally, I feel that indomethacin, a drug certainly not without side-effects, is probably the yardstick against which the drugs in this group should be measured. It has been used from the mid-1960s and both its benefits and complications are well known. Interestingly, it is one of the few anti-rheumatic drugs that has a higher concentration in the synovial fluid than in the blood; an obvious plus factor.

Recently the oral form has been modified to give a 'sustained release', which has the effect of giving a more prolonged and adequate level of the drug in the blood.

However, it is not without its side-effects, amongst which the most common are dyspepsia, headache, dizziness and tinnitus. For those patients prone to dyspepsia it can be given in suppository form. These side-effects occur in a small percentage of patients taking indomethacin, however, and do not present the major problems of phenylbutazone.

Is there any drug that does not cause dyspepsia?

In my experience one can never be 100 per cent dogmatic about anything in medicine because there will always be an exception. A drug called ibuprofen appears to have little in the way of side-effects on the gastro-intestinal tract and this would seem to be borne out by various clinical trials that have looked at this particular problem.

The drug itself also appears to have good anti-inflammatory effects, though no better than many of its rivals, some of the more common of which are: sulindac, tolmetin sodium, fenoprofen, naproxen, diclotenac, and ketoprofen.

There are many more and if you require further details please turn to the Drug Glossary on pp.145.

What place do steroids have in the treatment of rheumatoid arthritis?

In the 1950s, when steroids generally became available for use both in rheumatoid arthritis and other inflammatory diseases there was, as is often the case with a new drug, undue expectant euphoria over this new, 'miracle' cure. Some of this euphoria was warranted, for these new steroid drugs offered a completely new and dramatic therapeutic approach to the treatment of inflammatory disorders. As their use became more widespread, however, it became apparent that they had definite drawbacks and in some cases, serious side-effects that had, initially, not been predicted. Over the past 30 years, we have learned that, if used judiciously, steroids can be of great benefit in many diseases but that if used incorrectly they can worsen rather than help a disease process.

A word of warning may be useful here. Of late, there have been alarming reports that certain, unscrupulous people, not medically qualified, have been offering 'wonder cures' for those with arthritis, claiming their products and potions to be 'natural' remedies. In a few cases such remedies have been found to contain steroid preparations and have been taken unwittingly by the patient.

When should steroids be used in the treatment of rheumatoid arthritis?

Each patient is an individual case, and nowhere is this basic proposition more important to remember than in deciding whether to treat rheumatoid arthritis with steroids. Not only does the specific rheumatoid problem have to be individually assessed but the physician must also take into account the overall medical condition of his patient.

There are certain diseases that can be markedly exacerbated by steroids and although their use may be considered beneficial in terms of the patient's rheumatoid arthritis they may be contra-indicated if it is judged that they might make the patient's overall condition worse.

Before consideration is ever given to steroid therapy, most doctors would agree that an adequate trial of NSAIDs is mandatory. And not just one of the many drugs in this group, for, as I mentioned earlier, it is often a matter of trial and error before an anti-inflammatory drug can be found that controls the problem without too many unbearable side-effects.

Some doctors would advise that steroids should not be used until an adequate trial of either gold or penicillamine has been given. If a patient with more than one affected joint has not responded to either NSAIDs or a trial of gold and penicillamine, then oral steroids, normally in the form of prednisolone tablets may be started. Obviously, the dosage and the length of time that the treatment lasts is very much an individual matter but, in general terms, your doctor will use the lowest dose possible for the shortest period of time necessary to bring the rheumatoid problem under control.

Does age, occupation or lifestyle have any bearing on whether or not to use steroids?

As I shall describe later in my discussion on the benefits of exercise and physiotherapy, medication is used in conjunction with physical therapy to give affected joints the chance to benefit from the mobility these activities are designed to aid. In older patients, where physical exercise is either difficult or impossible, steroids may be given to maintain that patient's mobility rather than leaving him chairbound. Such therapy will also have to take account of this type of patient's general physical condition, bearing in mind the side-effects that I shall describe. Young patients, with juvenile rheumatoid arthritis, on the other hand, may have no alternative than to be treated with steroids, but growth can be affected if the therapy is not closely monitored.

Should steroids be used in children?

This is always a vexed question. Although these drugs can dampen down joint inflammation they can also have side-effects. These side-effects, which can, in some cases, result in growth problems, together with a suppression of the child's own steroid production must be weighed against the benefits they have of lessening the inflammation.

There is one specific area where steroids are invaluable, however, and that is in those few children whose hearts are affected by juvenile rheumatoid arthritis. In these cases steroids can have a dramatically beneficial effect in dampening down the inflammation of the heart muscle, known as myocarditis.

Can steroids be injected directly into joints?

Yes, they can, and, at first sight, bearing in mind the complications that can occur with taking steroids orally, this would seem to be a sensible way of administering the drug. Under certain circumstances, directly injecting steroids into joints has its advantages, especially if a patient's general rheumatoid status is well controlled by oral medication, leaving, perhaps, just one joint that has not responded to treatment.

In patients with a concurrent disease such as diabetes mellitus, which, as I shall describe, can be exacerbated by oral steroids, local joint injection can, in certain circumstances, get around this problem. Where joint mobility is required as part of a controlled programme of joint-exercising, a joint that has been resistant to other forms of medication can be made more mobile by a local steroid injection and so be more amenable to physical treatment.

Local steroid injections are not only given directly into the joints. In rheumatoid arthritis, the synovial linings of the tendons can become inflamed, causing pain, swelling and contractures. This problem can be locally treated by the use of steroid injections into the tendon sheaths. But, as with most forms of medication, there is another side to the coin. One of the problems with steroids is that far from inhibiting inflammation sometimes they can actually encourage infections – particularly if the injections are administered in anything but completely sterile conditions. They may also exacerbate an already infected joint that may have been misdiagnosed as a rheumatoid joint. In addition, there have been reports that increased joint destruction can result from such injections and that the bone surrounding the joints can become weakened.

How is the injection given into the joint and is it painful?

Before injecting the steroid your doctor will withdraw a variable amount of joint fluid to ensure that the rare possibility of joint infection has not been encountered. He will then feel the anatomical aspects of the joint by pressing gently on the skin surrounding the joint. Once he has precisely located the route that he is going to take he will pass the syringe needle through the skin and down to the joint. Apart from a slight prick as the needle pierces the skin you should feel no further pain or discomfort.

When will I feel the benefits of the injection?

Normally the beneficial effects of the injection – which will include a lessening of the swelling and of the pain together with an increase in joint mobility – will be noticed within three to four days. On average, the effects should last for about a month, by which time a natural recession in the joint's inflammation may well have begun to take place.

What are the main side-effects of steroids?

Normally when side-effects are mentioned they are in order of severity, but I feel that as far as steroids are concerned it is justifiable to make a distinction between side-effects that normally occur and can be described as 'acceptable' (though no side-effect can really be described as such) and those which can give rise to serious concern and which can sometimes lead to stopping the steroid treatment altogether.

What might be termed normally 'acceptable' side-effects are changes in hair texture, rather lighter sleeping than usual, an increased appetite, changes in menstruation, and slight mood swings.

As to the rather more serious side-effects the first is entirely in the control of both the doctor and his patient and it is important that every patient on steroids, whether taking them for arthritis or not, understands the following warning. When steroids are given they cause the body's own, internal supply of steroids, from the adrenal gland, to be reduced. If the steroids are then suddenly withdrawn, or if the patient forgets to take them, although the body can produce steroids to make up the deficit, such steroid production takes time, during which period the body is unable to protect itself from stress. At all times, therefore, you must carry with you a card that clearly states that you are taking steroids, the type and the dosage. Such cards are obtainable from your doctor.

You may think this absurd and that you will, after all, be in a position to tell anybody what you are taking, but don't forget the possibility that you may be involved in an accident and might be unconscious. Under these circumstances it is vital that the doctors looking after you know exactly what drugs you are taking, especially steroids, because they can give you steroids by injection, to substitute for your 'own' steroids.

What other side-effects can be expected from steroids?

As stated above, there will always be subtle changes that can be considered 'normal' and 'acceptable'. In order to treat your rheumatoid arthritis certain minor side-effects will be assumed to occur as a normal part of the treatment.

The following problems that can sometimes arise with steroid therapy, though not in the majority of cases, have to be weighed against the benefits that you are receiving from the steroid therapy. (In certain circumstances this will mean termination of the treatment.)

The skin becomes thin, cuts and bruises will take longer to heal than usual, and bruises will sometimes appear spontaneously. Facial features may fill out to give a more rounded appearance. In addition, hair may be lost from the head and, paradoxically, become prominent on the body. In children, growth – especially of the bones – can be stunted.

Fluid retention can also occur, causing swelling of the ankles and legs. This may sometimes even put an undue strain on the heart causing certain degrees of heart failure, normally noticed by increased breathlessness. Other side-effects of steroid therapy are increased weight gain and mood changes. In most cases these are not marked but sometimes they can be more exaggerated, with feelings of tremendous well-being (often described as 'being on a high') alternating with troughs of depression. It is important for both patient and family to be aware of this potential problem, because emotional changes of this sort can sometimes be misinterpreted as a separate psychological problem, not connected with arthritis or taking steroids.

Can taking steroids either cause or affect other illnesses?

In some patients, steroids can cause a particular sort of thinning of the bone known as osteoporosis (see p.43). This is more common in patients with arthritis and amongst the elderly, and your doctor will be very much on the look-out for this potential problem if you fall into these categories.

Another problem that is more common in patients with arthritis is a weakness of the muscles known as myopathy, and yet another that can either be initiated or exacerbated by steroids is diabetes mellitus. It is important, in this respect, that even if you do not have diabetes yet have a family history of the disease, you alert your doctor to this fact since a family history of the disease does slightly increase the likelihood of having diabetes induced by steroid medication.

One final point to bear in mind about steroids is that almost any infection can be masked if they are being taken, and so, if you are prone to infection, or suspect that you might have one seek your doctor's advice immediately.

With all these side-effects is it a good idea to take steroids in the first place?

Please don't be put off by the complications and side-effects of steroids that I have just mentioned. In all probability you will only experience the more minor side-effects. I have only gone to some lengths to tell you of the more serious problems to forewarn the small minority who will experience some of the rather more serious side-effects, so that they can be countered before they pose a serious risk to health.

What place does gold have in treating rheumatoid arthritis?

Gold injections will only be suggested by a consultant rheumatologist in selected cases where it is felt to be appropriate. It is a therapy that has to be carefully monitored, with regular attendance at hospital, and will normally follow a period of treatment with NSAIDs that has been unsuccessful in bringing the rheumatoid arthritis under control. But an acknowledged feature of gold therapy is the fact that there is inevitably a relatively large group of patients who will not respond to the treatment. And even with patients in whom beneficial effects are seen, a certain proportion will develop side-effects that will eventually mean having to stop the treatment altogether.

Historically, the use of gold was discovered accidentally. It was given to those with rheumatoid arthritis at the turn of the century in the belief that it was a cure for tuberculosis. (At that time it was thought that tuberculosis was one of the causes, if not the prime cause, of rheumatoid arthritis.) From its inception gold was seen to have a beneficial effect in some patients with rheumatoid arthritis – hence its present-day use in selected cases.

Is gold ever used to treat children?

Surprisingly, gold can help about 60 per cent of children with juvenile rheumatoid arthritis, though the various preparations of gold salts have to be administered by deep intramuscular injection. Although these drugs have side-effects, with careful monitoring these problems can be anticipated and the drugs withdrawn before any damage is done.

How is gold normally given?

Gold is administered by deep intramuscular injection. Initially there are a series of weekly doses, making up what is known as the loading dose. Thereafter, every fortnight or month, a maintenance dose is given, taking into account any side-effects and the state of the rheumatoid arthritis. It is important to remember that gold therapy does not have immediate benefits, taking an average of six months to produce a useful clinical response.

What side-effects are there from gold therapy?

Side-effects are a major drawback to gold therapy because, at one time or another, one or more of them are likely to be experienced by this form of treatment, though, paradoxically, the longer that the therapy is continued the less likely side-effects are to occur.

By far and away the most common problems are seen with the skin ranging from a barely perceptible skin rash, with minimal itching, through rather more noticeable forms of allergic skin reactions to a severe form of skin allergy. Inflammatory changes around the gums and in the mouth, causing soreness with eating and drinking, are other annoying side-effects. Problems can also occur with the kidney as well as with the cells in the blood concerned with blood-clotting (platelets).

The only treatment for such side-effects is to stop the therapy, though in certain cases this can be recommenced at a lower dosage.

Are there any other drugs with a similar action to gold but without its side-effects?

One drug you might have come across is penicillamine. Like gold it is not an anti-inflammatory drug, but, rather, acts by slowing down the progress of rheumatoid arthritis. Like gold, however, it has side-effects. Chief amongst these are dyspepsia and loss of taste, though other problems include damage to the kidney, skin rashes and the development of a number of rare syndromes which are all connected by the common thread of allergy.

There does not, on the whole, appear to be any advantage in using penicillamine in preference to gold though, of course, in an appropriate patient, in whom gold has caused unwanted reactions, penicillamine may be a substitute with, hopefully, none of its side-effects.

Is it true that certain drugs for the treatment of malaria are used in the treatment of rheumatoid arthritis?

Yes, this certainly is true, the drugs in question being chloroquine and hydroxychloroquine. As with gold therapy, the decision to start treatment with these drugs will only be taken by your specialist rheumatologist, and a sometimes lengthy period of time may sometimes elapse before any noticeably beneficial effects are felt.

There are side-effects associated with these drugs, too, the most common of which is dyspepsia. But by far the most serious problem that can be caused by taking these anti-malarial drugs is in the eye, where the retina can be affected. If you are given a course of these drugs, therefore, you will have your eyes examined before and during treatment. The eye examinations are entirely painless and will involve testing colour vision as well as the field of vision, though the eye specialist will also look at the retina directly to ensure that no damage is being done. As long as these eye examinations are regularly carried out there is barely any risk to your vision while you are undergoing this type of treatment.

Do copper bracelets help arthritis?

From a strictly scientific point of view there is no evidence whatsoever that copper bracelets have any effect on the disease.

However, there is no doubt about the fact that in some cases such bracelets *do* give sufferers great relief, and it would be a brave doctor who dissuaded his patients from wearing them. Wearing such bracelets certainly does no harm and, under these circumstances, if they do give symptomatic relief, and help you, wear them.

Are there any dietary considerations I should be following to help my arthritic condition?

Certainly. In general terms, there is one thing that you can do and that is to set yourself what you consider to be, for you, a sensible and attainable weight. This is particularly important if you suffer from osteoarthritis of the hip. The less weight your diseased joints have to bear, the fewer will be the consequences of the arthritic condition. Losing weight will not cure the arthritis but it will at least help to mitigate the problem.

I am not going to go into the vexed question of dieting here because I believe that there has been more nonsense written about this subject that any other subject connected with health. It seems to me that one of the essential points that the prophetic dietitians who rite these books always seem to overlook is the fact that each of us is different, that we are all individuals, born with a certain individual programmed body shape and weight, and that we each have specific appetite requirements, as well as a taste for certain foods and a dislike of others. Whenever we read a book on dieting, we are told first what weight we should be and secondly, that we should eat specific foods, in specific quantities to attain that weight. If we were all the same, this would present no problem. But we aren't.

Let's use some common sense here. We all know when we are overweight and we all know how to lose weight by cutting down on the food that we are eating and doing a little more exercise.

But, what about specific diets, I hear you ask? I have looked long and hard at all the claims and counter-claims and at the various suggestions that have cropped up, over the years, and, to be honest, there really are no specific considerations to follow, in terms of, say, excluding particular items from your diet. There is, however, one exception to this and that is the arthritis due to gout which, in the main, can be brought on by too much alcohol or too much food (or, indeed too much exercise). It is equally important to realize, on the other hand, that by starving yourself, you can sometimes induce an attack of gout. In cases of gouty arthritis, therefore, be guided by what your doctor advises you to eat and drink.

What treatment is available to help eyes affected by rheumatoid arthritis?

There are several ways in which arthritis can affect the eyes and I shall discuss their treatment in turn.

Firstly, 'dry eyes' a condition which can give a gritty sensation on blinking together with pain and irritation. Since the condition is due to defective tear production (see p.22) it is treated by the frequent application of bland eye drops – in effect, tear substitutes. If frequent applications of these tear substitutes are inadequate, further measures can be taken, such as blocking the tear ducts to prevent the tears that are already formed from flowing away too easily.

Secondly, redness. This must be taken very seriously and not simply put down to conjunctivitis. For, although if you have arthritis you are just as likely as anybody else to get conjunctivitis, there are many eye problems you can get that may be mistaken for conjunctivitis, but which may in fact be quite different and will require entirely different treatments. One of these conditions is known as iritis which is actually inflammation within the eye Treatment consists of applications of steroid drops together with drops that dilate the pupil. This may have to be continued for some weeks before the inflammation begins to subside.

Two other diseases that can often be mistaken for conjunctivitis involve the white of the eye. They are episcleritis and scleritis and have been dealt with on p.23. Both should be assessed and treated by an eye specialist.

Can thermal therapy be used in rheumatoid arthritis?

For centuries, it has been known that thermal therapy, or applications of either heat or cold, on or near particularly painful sites of rheumatic disease can give rapid and welcome relief. But, despite the fact that these simple truths have been well recognized from Roman times, there is still no completely satisfactory explanation as to how pain relief should be modified in this way.

It is quite true that, by applying local heat, a certain increase in blood flow occurs to a particular part, but this increased blood supply is demonstrated most easily in the skin and superficial tissues, whereas most of the pain from rheumatoid arthritis undoubtedly comes from pain receptors in and around the affected joints.

As well as this somewhat anomalous theory of increased blood flow there is also the problem of explaining how the application of cold compresses, which also give relief but which can be shown to decrease blood flow to an area, exert their effect.

The fact that symptoms can be relieved by either heat or cold suggests that the relief is somehow bound up with a change in temperature rather than a specific temperature itself.

Thermal therapy works in two, closely connected, ways. First, by itself it can give relief of pain and a general sense of well being as well as allowing for a greater amount of joint mobility. Secondly, due to these benefits, it can greatly assist in the mobilization of joints as part of an organized programme of exercise that we shall be discussing in a later section. Following exercise, it can bring a soothing relaxation to muscles and joints.

Do remember, as you read on, that some of the following treatments may not be appropriate for your particular problem so consult your doctor before embarking upon any of them.

An important point in this respect is to remember that if a joint is acutely inflamed the application of too much heat, whether combined with exercise or not, may result in further damage.

Skin can also be quite badly damaged by excessive application of either heat or cold. Be careful, therefore, not to use excessive thermal therapy – especially if treating yourself at home.

The most common forms of thermal therapy are: moist heat, wax applications, deep heat and cold therapy.

Whichever form you choose, if applying the treatment at home, organize yourself and the apparatus so that everything is to hand, allowing for as much relaxation as possible, for relaxation is just as important as the thermal therapy, itself.

Finally, a useful way of using thermal therapy may be to

combine it with hydrotherapy. Perhaps the easiest way to do this is a warm bath. Simple, but used correctly, warm baths can be extremely beneficial.

What is moist heat and how should it be used?

Moist heat, as opposed to dry heat (normally given in the form of infra-red radiation) can be given in many forms, the most convenient probably being moist heat packs. These are simple to use, easy to apply, clean and non-messy. Each pack contains silica gel. This is warmed with hot water and the pack or packs are applied to the particular joints for up to about half an hour. As long as these warm packs are kept within safe temperature limits they can be used up to three times daily.

A modern alternative to moist heat is to apply a soft, heated, electric pad to the affected joints. But remember that you probably have a somewhat larger and modified pad of your own – your electric blanket.

Used judiciously, electric blankets can bring immense relief in beds which otherwise, if cold, can exacerbate a general arthritic problem.

Do wax baths have a place in the thermal treatment of rheumatoid arthritis?

Used from about the turn of the century paraffin wax baths have stood the test of time though with more modern types of thermal therapy available today they are not being used as much as they used to be.

There are two ways of giving this form of treatment. The paraffin wax can be applied locally, with a brush, or the affected part of the body, such as the hand or wrist, can be directly immersed into the warm wax.

Although this therapy has, of necessity, to be given under

medical supervision it can be done at home. A word of warning, however. Paraffin baths can ignite so if using them do bear this fire hazard in mind.

What is deep heat therapy?

The forms of thermal therapy that I have so far discussed are known, in general terms, as superficial thermal therapy. But there is another form of heat treatment known as deep heat treatment. And, as with other forms of heat treatment, the precise way in which it brings about its effects is not known.

The use of deep heat treatment is largely confined to patients who do not suffer from arthritic diseases as such but who have injured or sprained ligaments and muscles surrounding a joint.

The most commonly used form of deep heat therapy is ultrasound and, less commonly, diathermy treatment. The effectiveness of both these forms of treatment lies in their ability to reduce muscular spasm in the muscles surrounding the affected joints.

Can cold therapy help rheumatoid arthritis?

It is well known by sportsmen, in particular, that following a painful injury, such as a cricket ball hitting a wrist, the application of a cold spray such as ethyl chloride can greatly reduce the pain from the injured spot. The scientific foundation as to how this works is not known though part of the efficacy of this treatment is due to the numbing of the pain receptors in and around the injured part.

Some patients with rheumatoid arthritis can be helped by the application of judiciously placed ice packs over the inflamed joints. Some experts advise alternating this cold therapy with some form of warm therapy, though this form of 'alternating' thermal therapy is rarely used.

What importance is attached to correct posture and walking with arthritis?

Posture, whether you are sitting, lying or walking is always important, even if you haven't got arthritis. If you *do* have arthritis, it is particularly important, both throughout the day and during those periods when you are doing the specific exercises that your doctor and physiotherapist have prescribed for you. I shall be dealing with these exercises later. Meanwhile, I should like to talk, in basic terms, about posture.

One of the most characteristic and annoying features of rheumatoid arthritis is morning stiffness. Although this problem cannot be completely eliminated, it can be reduced by attention to posture while either resting or sleeping in bed.

Now let me spell out a few 'dos and dont's'. It is sometimes very tempting when pain and stiffness of the joints in the legs is troublesome, to position your knees in a bent position with a pillow to support them. Although this can give temporary relief, in the long run it can create more problems than it solves in that increased joint immobility and contraction and rigidity of the surrounding tissues and muscles can occur. Therefore, never, when lying in bed, support bent knees by pillows.

And, talking of pillows, try not to use too many to support your head and neck – one should be sufficient.

Now, as to the bed itself. Later on in the book, I shall be going in detail into the precise bedroom arrangements that are of practical value, but at this stage I would emphasize that a firm mattress should be used rather than a somewhat more comfortable mattress that might lack adequate support. There are plenty of firm mattresses that combine rigidity with comfort and if your sleeping partner does not like a firm mattress it is quite possible to get double beds with one half that has a firm mattress and the other half that has a less rigid one.

Then there is standing. This can be an ordeal for both those with rheumatoid arthritis and osteoarthritis for not only can standing put uneven weight on joints such as the knees and in the feet, but it can also be complicated by, in some cases, shortening of the legs, which often accompanies these conditions. The main thing is to try and stand as straight as possible, though without exaggerating this to the point of discomfort. Try and keep your shoulders as far back as possible and at the same time try to prevent your neck from bending too far forwards.

When sitting, apply the same criteria to your chair as you will have done to your bed: Firmness, but not to the point of discomfort. A firm, supportive back to a chair can go a long way to helping chronic back problem.

Allow yourself to move in the chair and don't sit for too long in any one position. Also, make sure that you do not sink back into your chair in a position that will then be difficult to get up from.

One final word, about posture when lifting heavy objects. Never allow your back to take the weight by bending it while lifting. Always bend your knees and hips when picking up any sort of object from the floor.

In what precise way can arthritis affect my walking?

Walking is one of those activities that comes so naturally that it is taken for granted. It is not until ambulatory problems arise that walking, as an activity, is consciously thought about.

I should like to begin by briefly examining what normal walking entails before going into the problems of walking that arthritis can throw up.

So, what parts of our bodies are involved in the process of walking? At first sight, it would seem that walking simply involves putting one leg in front of the other. In a limited sense, this is true. But, as I shall describe, not only does the pelvis play an integral part in the propulsion of the lower limbs, so also do the shoulders and the arms – both as part of the overall forward motion of the body as well as in the overall balance.

Having introduced the word balance, I should also like to show how arthritis, in particular, can pose problems to the body's normal balance mechanism, because the way in which we are able to balance is one of the most intricate functions that we carry out subconsciously. By seeing where we are in space, our eyes can give our brains useful, basic data in orientating ourselves to the horizon and in relation to the ground and other objects around us. Within our ears we have a very sophisticated balancing mechanism that is, in effect, self-righting: it allows us, whether we are sitting or running at speed, to alter our posture and stance so that we do not lose balance.

Finally, as an integral part of our mechanism, which includes the eyes and the inner ear, is the third important component that we possess to maintain our balance. Surrounding the joints are specialized nerve endings (called proprioceptors) that are, in effect, miniature spirit levels, constantly passing messages to our brains telling us where exactly each and every joint is.

So you can appreciate that if certain joints are inflamed due to rheumatoid arthritis, this delicate balancing mechanism can be partially compromised. Although this is never a major problem, it *can* add to the other problems thrown up by rheumatoid arthritis and osteoarthritis as regards walking.

So, apart from balance, what is involved in normal walking?

First there is the supporting, or 'stance' phase. This begins when the heel of one leg touches the ground and the leg itself begins to support the weight of the body. At this moment, the hip joint, which has been extended, turns slightly inward, which allows the walker to carry on forwards, in a straight line. Then the hip joint has to tilt outwards, on the supporting leg to allow the pelvis to give the other leg, the swinging leg, the lift necessary to swing forwards. While all this is going on at the top of the leg, the knee joint is being extended while, at the ankle joint, there is flexion followed by extension. And this isn't all, for, in the foot the numerous small joints are all playing their part in taking the weight of the supporting leg.

Once the supporting leg has done its job, it becomes the swinging leg as the next, 'swing' phase begins. At the hip joint there is flexion together with an outwards rotation, at the knee joint there is flexion, and at the ankle joint there is extension followed by flexion.

But the details of all this don't really matter. The important point is that walking can be seen to be a very complex matter and I'm sure that you can appreciate that a problem in just one single joint can cause the complex processes to become disrupted.

So, can a doctor tell where the problem lies simply by watching somebody with a walking difficulty?

Yes, certainly.

But I don't want to go into great technical detail about the diagnostic niceties involved. Suffice it to say that your doctor will want to see you walking. When you do this for him, don't try to walk correctly – just let him see your 'normal' gait, for this will help him diagnose the problem. I should, by the way of illustration, like to take a common clinical problem to show you how useful the study of gait is. The problem is called metatarsalgia.

What is metatarsalgia?

Metatarsalgia is a term used to describe pain arising from the foot, and in particular, pain arising from a specific series of small bones in the middle of the foot – the bones that take the weight of the whole body.

To avoid excessive pain, patients with metatarsalgia tend to alter their normal walking pattern, showing an unwillingness to flex the foot and to extend both the knee as well as the hip. Also, the muscles surrounding these under-utilized joints can fall into disuse and become weakened, causing a generalized weakness of the whole leg.

So you can see how just one small painful area can upset the whole balance of a normal gait. This is, of course, just one example, but every joint involved in walking can give rise to similar and unique gait problems. And, as with so many of these gait problems, once the diagnosis has been accurately made (and this is sometimes difficult if two or more joints are involved when trying to pinpoint the initiating culprit) simple treatment can normally be most effective.

In the case of metatarsalgia a metatarsal support can be fitted inside the shoe, allowing redistribution of the weight formerly taken by the metatarsal area and now supplied by a greater proportion of the foot, as a whole.

What other aids are there that can help with walking and how should they be used?

I should like to begin by dealing with some general principles because it is particularly important that one arthritic problem is not solved at the expense of another. For instance, it may seem sensible to use a stick to relieve weight-bearing on an arthritic hip, but this might create problems in the hand, wrist, elbow or shoulder joint of the arm that are taking the weight, through the stick, that the diseased hip formerly took.

Another point to bear in mind is that some assistive devices, due either to their complexity or incorrect use, can result in excessive weight-bearing on vulnerable joints, thus causing more problems than they solve.

Common sense is therefore important when choosing walking aids. A typical example of this is shoes. Although in some cases there is a need for specially made orthopaedic shoes, in the main, as long as the shoe is sturdy, well constructed, fits snugly on the foot and gives comfortable support it will normally be perfectly adequate. In rather more serious cases, external supports such as splints and braces may be necessary and I shall deal with these in greater detail in my discussions on rest and exercise.

For now, I should like to concentrate on some specific, basic aids that can help with walking.

Firstly, walking sticks. Before choosing your stick, make sure that it is the correct length. Wooden sticks can easily be cut to the length you need, while the more modern, light aluminium varieties can normally be easily adjusted by extension or recession of the lower end of the stick's two sections. As far as the handle of the stick is concerned, there are a number of different shapes to accommodate any problems that might occur with grip or mis-shapen hands. Make sure that there is a secure rubber end to the stick to avoid any chance of it slipping when you place it on the ground.

A number of more sophisticated walking aids such as walking frames, both with and without wheels, are now readily available. Ask your doctor and physiotherapist which model they advise for you. Similarly, professional advice will also be necessary if you use crutches, in order that you get the full benefit that such supports can give. When walking with crutches, remember that balance is all-important.

Always watch where you place the tips of your crutches: slippery floors, thick, pile carpets or rough ground can all be potential hazards.

Widening your stance will normally be of great value in increasing the ability to balance. But, remember, there are specific techniques for walking with crutches and your physiotherapist will demonstrate to you the method best suited to your particular problem.

Finally, wheelchairs. Always bear in mind that the most expensive is not necessarily the best. Decide what your specific wheelchair needs are. Write these down on a piece of paper and then decide which make and model will be best suited for your needs. Points to look out for are: compactness of storage both at home and in a car, ease of movement around your environment, detachable sides, and weight – remembering that your helper may have to do the lifting.

Information on mechanical aids in the home is given on pp.128-135.

What exercises can be done to help rheumatoid arthritis?

Again I should like to begin by laying down some overall principles and guidelines, and then go on to describe individual exercises and specific examples of how they may be used.

The most important thing to remember is that this is a very

individual problem. Every patient should be guided by their own doctor in conjunction with their physiotherapist. Before a programme of exercises is even drawn up, it is essential to know what the patient's individual home conditions are as well as the nature of his or her daily activities. It is important that the exercise programme be built into this pattern so that it is disrupted as little as possible.

Side by side with exercise is the important principle of adequate rest. The amount and proportion of exercise set against rest are very much a matter of individual assessment.

How much rest should I take?

As I have said previously, there is a whole spectrum of problems that can arise in rheumatoid arthritis, from slight inflammation of a single joint to a severe debilitating disease involving not only the joints but the whole body.

For minor problems, common sense is the rule. If you have used the affected joint or joints excessively, take a rest; sit down; allow things to settle down and you yourself will know, from experience, when you are up to resuming your usual tasks. If the rheumatic condition is causing a generalized problem, your doctor and physiotherapist will be monitoring the situation and giving specific guidelines as to rest and exercise.

But what about those occasions when you have a flare-up in a number of joints or an excessive exacerbation in one joint? Should you put everything down and just retire to bed?

Current thought would certainly advise taking a rest and, if it makes you feel better, going to bed. Time in bed should be kept to a minimum, however, since the consequent joint stiffness that inevitably follows too long a rest in one position can progress to joint immobility, with or without contractures.

What are contractures and can they be prevented?

Although many people associate this word with overt deformity, it is really used to describe limitation of movement. A common misconception is that contractures are somehow due to muscle shrinkage. This is incorrect, for the basic problem lies in the fibrous tissue which is an integral part of the ligaments and tendons in the areas of contracture.

It is the loss of joint mobility that is the cause of contractures, though it may not be the actual joint itself that is at fault but rather the tendons that act upon the muscle which give the joint its mobility.

Contractures are fairly uncommon as a part of arthritic disease and even in cases where they begin to appear they can normally be prevented from progressing. There is a variety of treatments, but all follow the same basic principle in that they encourage passive movements in the form of painless exercise designed to prevent the contractures from developing and progressing. Such exercises are not painful – in fact, a cardinal rule is that they should not be conducted if there is any pain.

Your doctor or physiotherapist will advise whether or not the affected joints should be surrounded with protective splints in order to avoid the painful muscle contractures that sometimes go hand in hand with joint immobility.

What is splinting and why is it used?

As mentioned earlier, a very fine balance has to be kept between, on the one hand, sufficient exercise of an affected joint and, on the other, adequate rest. What splinting does is to support an affected joint, resting that joint but also, to a limited extent, allowing it to exercise.

Splints can also be applied to immobilize the joints while they are resting. This is done to relieve pain and to stop the inflammatory process proceeding. And, as a consequence, diminishes any deformities that might arise. Sometimes splints that are applied while the joint is resting have a different purpose. If, for instance, a contracture has occurred, such splinting can try and modify the contracture and try to correct the deformed anatomy.

Splints may also be applied during periods of activity to protect the joints. In short, it is important to realize, when talking about splinting, that there are specific splints for specific purposes and to appreciate whether the splinting is designed for mobilization or periods of rest.

Finally, it is important, if you are undergoing splinting treatment, to have regular assessments. For one of the hallmarks of rheumatic disease is the way in which it changes. Thus, although a specific splint may initially be fulfilling a purpose, it may, if not checked, become counter-productive. Regular check-ups from your physiotherapist are very important.

What forms, in general, do the exercises you have mentioned take?

There are three basic forms of exercise. One type is isometric The essential thing about these exercises is that (although arthritis is present in the joints) the joints, themselves, are not moved, but rather, the muscles, acting upon the joint, are contracted and relaxed, by the patient. This form of exercise can either be done at home or in a physiotherapy department.

Another type of exercise is where the joint is moved by the patient but where the patient is helped in the movement, by a physiotherapist, a friend or a family member.

Finally, there is the most common group of exercises – those done entirely by the patient, but, again, performed to a general schedule advised by the doctor and physiotherapist.

Any of these three forms of exercise can be performed depending on the state of the rheumatoid arthritis. But I must emphasize that when and for how long they are used is very much an individual matter. Certainly, under normal circumstances, they are contraindicated if pain is either present or induced by the exercises.

One useful tip while doing exercises is to have on, at the same time, the television, radio or a cassette – this can make the whole process so much more pleasant.

In addition to the general forms of exercises just described, there is another type of exercise that the physiotherapist might do for you. This comprises the various forms of passive stretching exercises that the physiotherapist will undertake in an attempt to give you more joint mobility and to stop such deformities as contractures occurring.

Don't worry about these – physiotherapists are very experienced people. There may be slight pain but it will not be intolerable. Eventually, once you are used to your set of exercises, you will find how easily they can be slipped into your daily routine.

Although exercises cannot cure the arthritic problem, they can certainly keep the disease at bay.

Are there any conditions under which it is best to do these exercises?

As I have continually emphasized, every patient is an individual and under these circumstances it is difficult to generalize. However, under certain circumstances, thermal therapy can be applied before the exercise routine is begun and may, in certain circumstances, greatly facilitate the exercise programme.

When is the best time for me to do my exercises?

When do you feel least tired and when are your joints at their best? Answer this question and you will probably have named the time best suited for you, though with obvious limitations. If, for example, you feel at your best at work, you might not always find it practically possible to carry out a programme of exercises.

As most people find that they feel at their best in the mornings it is probably a good idea to do your exercises just after getting out of bed. There is, however, another school of thought that contends that a better night's sleep is gained if exercises are done just before retiring. In short, then, it is very much a matter of personal choice.

What part does physiotherapy have to play in rehabilitating children with juvenile rheumatoid arthritis?

Physiotherapy is extremely important in the treatment of these children.

The key word is balance. On the one hand, rest – both total body rest and also rest of the affected joints – must be adequate, especially in the acute phase. Set against this, joint mobility must be sustained in order that fixed joints and contractures do not occur and also that the muscles supporting these joints do not become weak.

Combined with the physiotherapy, splinting the affected joints to protect them is sometimes necessary, at certain stages of the disease process. Here again, there must be a fine balance between immobilization by splints for adequate joint protection and mobilization with or without splinting, to prevent permanent joint deformity.

Can massage help my arthritis?

There are many theories as to how massage works but, as yet, there is no convincing scientific explanation of its undoubted benefits, one of which is that it appears to do little or no harm. It is said that massage to certain areas has an effect on the local blood flow. Whatever the reasons for its success, massage can definitely be a useful adjunct in the treatment of arthritis though it is important to receive it only from a fully qualified masseur. Seek your doctor's advice on this matter.

Could you give some examples of how exercise and rest can be used to advantage in rheumatoid arthritis?

I think that for a number of reasons it would be useful to look in detail at how these principles of exercise and rest can be applied to the hand and wrist. I must emphasize, however, that the descriptions which follow are purely illustrative examples. Do not carry out the various procedures that I describe without first consulting your doctor or physiotherapist, for they may not be applicable in your particular situation.

Let us imagine that one morning you wake up to find that your hand, known to have rheumatoid arthritis, is acutely painful, swollen and that movements are only made with undue difficulty. Obviously, you will go to your doctor and he will either increase your present medication or prescribe something more efficacious. He will then ask you to attend your physiotherapist with, in general terms, a plan of physical therapy. This, in the initial and acute stages, will probably mean some form of splinting.

As described earlier splinting has many uses. In the acute phase of rheumatoid flare-up, it not only helps the hand to maintain a degree of function, but is also perhaps the most efficient way of making it comfortable. In this phase the splint is worn continually, being removed only for exercises, which normally take the form of assisted exercises described above. With the passage of time, the acute phase will be controlled by a combination of medication, splinting, exercise, rest and probably some form of thermal therapy.

When this phase is over you will probably feel inclined to relax your guard and simply go back to relying on medication. Taking this line is usually incorrect, however, for it is precisely during this quiescent, or dormant, phase that the characteristic deformities of rheumatoid arthritis can occur. The way to prevent this is to use a combination of splinting (to prevent deformity), and exercises (to maintain and increase joint mobility).

There is a particular type of splint that can be used at the wrist during the quiescent phase that will not only prevent deformities but will also allow mobility of the joint without excessive pain.

At the same time, it will give support to the wrist and, as a consequence, to the whole hand, when lifting or weight-bearing. Splinting in the quiescent phase may take many forms, there being special splints for the various joints in the hand, but all have the same function.

As well as splinting exercise is also important during this quiescent stage. For the hand and wrist, the best forms of exercises are both the isometric and the active exercises, though the latter should not be overdone, in the early phases. Also, as I indicated earlier, some of the exercises can be made easier by the concurrent use of thermal therapy. It is important to emphasize and reiterate that while this quiescent phase lasts the exercises should be maintained. But before embarking on them always consult your doctor and physiotherapist to ensure that they are safe for you.

What is hydrotherapy and how can it be used in rheumatoid arthritis?

Hydrotherapy is the treatment of any condition – arthritic or otherwise – by the use of water. In the case of arthritis this is invariably warm water.

The benefits of a warm bath were mentioned earlier, in my discussion of thermal therapy. It is well known that for anybody whose body has received a pounding there is no better way to relax than by wallowing in a nice hot bath. But one feature that makes warm water therapy so useful to arthritic patients is the fact that exercises done immediately after immersion in hot water are invariably more easily carried out.

A further plus factor of water therapy arises from its property of buoyancy. Of necessity, much less strain is put upon a joint while the bones, muscles and ligaments surrounding the joint are supported by the buoyancy of the water.

How is hydrotherapy given?

Hydrotherapy can, of course, be received in an ordinary bath. Even though this may seem simple, however, do be guided by your physiotherapist because exercises incorrectly done, even with the help of the buoyancy of the water, can in some cases, do more harm than good.

Nowadays, many more hydrotherapy pools are coming into their own. These are normally situated in departments of physiotherapy and when using them you will automatically be under the guidance of a physiotherapist. Such centres are still few and far between, however, and you may find that a very satisfactory substitute is your local swimming pool.

There are a series of basic hydrotherapy exercises that can be carried out, although you should always consult your doctor to ensure that the exercises that you propose to carry out in the pool will not overtax you or, in some cases, be detrimental to your programme of rehabilitation.

If you use a public swimming pool don't forget two essential facts: the pool's water will be much cooler than is normally used in most physiotherapy departments and, as a consequence, joint movement may not be so easy; also be especially careful not to over-exercise. If you carry out exercises unsupervised, this can easily happen.

Can surgery ever help an arthritic condition?

In recent years, surgery has begun to play an increasingly important part in the overall treatment of both rheumatoid arthritis and osteoarthritis. Up to now, in this section on general orthodox therapy for arthritis, I have concentrated mainly on rheumatoid arthritis, despite the fact that more people are diagnosed with osteoarthritis.

At this stage, however, I should like to concentrate on osteoarthritis and, in particular, on osteoarthritis of the hip, which, in certain circumstances, lends itself to surgical correction with a high degree of satisfactory results.

In discussing surgery for the osteoarthritic hip, I would like to use this both as a general and specific illustrative example of what you, as a patient, should expect, from the initial stages of diagnosis, through the operative period and into the post-operative period of physiotherapy.

How is osteoarthritis of the hip joint diagnosed?

The first essential fact to realize is that osteoarthritis of the hip joint is a slowly evolving problem and it can take many years before the problem is serious enough to warrant surgery.

Pain is invariably present to some degree but it is not necessarily localized in the region of the hip joint. It can, for instance, be felt in the knee or back, though most commonly the pain is experienced in the groin and in the front of the thigh.

As I mentioned, earlier, stiffness is a common problem of both rheumatoid arthritis and osteoarthritis. Characteristically, with osteoarthritis of the hip, getting up out of a chair and immediately walking is often not possible and many patients will describe a period during which they need time to 'get going'.

Other consequences of this stiffness result in difficulty in carrying out routine activities such as tying shoe-laces and cutting nails. And then, of course, there are the problems of walking. These occur mainly because of increasing pain, that necessarily restricts the walker. But a further factor causing walking problems is what is known as 'apparent shortening' of the affected leg. When measured against its partner, the leg of the affected hip may be found to be 'shorter'. This is often due to spasm of some of the muscles surrounding the hip joint which causes the pelvis to tilt to the side of the osteoarthritic hip. As a consequence of this, the vertebral column can become misshapen, a condition called scoliosis.

So, when you go to your doctor you may confront him with a variety of symptoms such as pain in various regions, problems with getting up from chairs, perhaps a limp together with an abnormal stance and, in certain circumstances, a slight back deformity.

How will the doctor treat my osteoarthritis of the hip?

The first thing your doctor will do will be to take a complete history of all your symptoms and when they began to appear. He will then discuss with you the sort of problems they are causing and will go on to examine your hip, probably asking you to walk a few paces so that he can observe any gait problems. Your stance will then be examined. When your doctor does this, he will be looking for any tilt of your pelvis, and any back-related problems as well as signs of 'apparent' leg shortening. Then, while you lie on the examining couch, the various movements of your hip joint will be assessed. Do not be surprised if your doctor then examines other joints as well as giving you a general examination. All this is part of a normal work-up of the complete clinical picture, for, at this stage, your doctor will be necessarily considering the possibility of perhaps rheumatoid arthritis of the hip joint and will be looking for evidence for and against this hypothesis.

Following the examination, your doctor will request that X-rays be taken of the hip joint and ask you to return when the results are through.

What will my doctor do for me when I subsequently consult him?

Much will, of course, depend on the results of your X-rays, together with the clinical findings that your doctor will have made at the initial examination.

Let us assume that your doctor makes the diagnosis of osteo-arthritis of the hip and tells you that it is at an early stage. What will be done for you?

First, the general nature of osteoarthritis will be explained to you. Then, unless you are fairly exceptional, your doctor will tactfully consult his notes and tell you what you really already knew: that you are overweight and that a course of dieting and weight reduction are necessary.

Weight reduction, especially in osteoarthritis of the hip, can greatly help the problem. The less weight that the hip has to support, the more slowly the osteoarthritis will develop and, with the reduction in the weight that the joint has to bear, so will the pain be lessened.

Your doctor will also advise you on the amount of rest and exercise that you should take, taking into account your age and general physical condition. Having advised you on these general matters he will then turn to more specific measures that can be prescribed to help you. The first of these will be drugs to both ease the pain and help the condition. You will recall that when discussing the treatment of rheumatoid arthritis I mentioned a group of drugs that were loosely categorized as the 'non-steroidal anti-inflammatory drugs' (NSAIDs). Your doctor will probably give you a trial of one of these (see Drug Glossary, pp.145) as well as a pain-killing drug such as paracetamol for particularly painful exacerbations of the problem.

Then will come the question of walking aids, the choice of which is very much a matter of personal preference and practicality.

Finally, your general practitioner will advise you about not causing undue stress and trauma to the hip, as in, for instance, the injudicious pursuit of sporting interests.

At what stage will I be able to have an operation on my hip?

The decision to operate on a hip with osteoarthritis is never a straightforward one, for many factors have to be taken into account.

Normally, the measures prescribed by your general practitioner will, for a variable length of time, help, if not completely solve, the problem.

However, there will always be a group of patients who find that either the pain from their arthritic hip is unbearable and is not being controlled by drugs, or that their normal activities, including their work or leisure, are being seriously affected by the problem and they feel that something more needs to be done.

Again, your doctor may feel that the effects of your problem (abnormal gait, together with all the secondary effects such as back problems) that can be caused by an arthritic hip can only be improved by an operation.

Under these circumstances he will then feel that it is time to send you to a specialist, who will normally be an orthopaedic surgeon.

Will the orthopaedic surgeon operate straight away?

The answer to this question is probably not. When you see your surgeon for the first time he will go over your symptoms and examine you in very much the same way as your doctor will have already done. As he carries out his detailed examinations, together with further X-rays, the question uppermost in his mind will be when is the best time for you, as his patient, to undergo hip surgery. Apart from the specific judgement that he will come to concerning the state of your arthritic hip he will have to assess your general condition and whether a hip operation will be successful in your particular case. He must also ascertain whether you have any other medical conditions such as heart disease or diabetes mellitus that may complicate both the operative and post-operative phases, or chest and breathing problems that may pose the anaesthetist a problem.

On the other hand, he will also know the benefits to be gained from an operation. So, although he may advise putting off surgery for a few more months, eventually, when he feels that the time is right, you will be called into hospital for an operation.

What does hip replacement surgery involve?

In answering this question I shall briefly mention the general procedures that you would normally expect on admission to hospital. I am doing this because, in a number of cases, people with osteoarthritis of the hip are otherwise healthy, and it is probably their first admission to hospital for a major operation.

On admission to your ward, your details will normally be taken by one of the nursing staff. At present, the nursing profession are introducing a system called 'the nursing process'. This is an excellent practice for it encourages individual nurses to, for as much time as is possible, nurse and be responsible for a specific patient during his or her stay in hospital. This will mean that for much of the time you will have the same nurse looking after you – a state of affairs that undoubtedly has many benefits.

Once you have been admitted, you will then be seen by the house surgeon, the junior hospital doctor who works with and assists your consultant. The house surgeon will take down your medical history, even though this will probably have been done in the outpatients' department and also by the nursing staff. You may feel that this is an unnecessary duplication of work but, overall, this system of checks and double checks will ensure that by the time you are taken to theatre the correct patient will be about to have the correct operation on the correct leg.

You will then be visited by your anaesthetist who will examine you, specifically for potential chest and cardiac problems so that these may be avoided during the operation. The next morning you will probably be seen by your consultant, on his ward round. He will give you a final examination and make sure that all the other members of staff have completed their appointed tasks.

What happens on operation day?

In case of anaesthetic problems you will have received 'nil by mouth' for some hours prior to the operation. About an hour before the operation you will be given your pre-medication. This consists of a sedative drug as well as a drug that dries up the natural secretions of your chest that makes the procedure of anaesthetizing you all the easier. You will then be taken to theatre, where your anaesthetist will check that he is about to anaesthetize the correct patient. Following a small prick on the back of your hand you will next wake up in your bed with a new hip.

What actually happens during the operation?

In essence, your surgeon will make an incision through the skin over your hip and will then dissect his way down to the hip joint. Once he has isolated the joint he will then begin the hip replacement.

First, he will remove the top of the femur or thigh bone, which will invariably show the marked irregularities of osteoarthritis. He will then insert into the pelvic bone a plastic cup that will eventually take the metallic artificial ball which takes the place of the diseased top of the femur. The plastic cup is attached to the pelvic bone by a special cement. Once it is in position, the metallic ball is inserted into the hip bone, its shaft being inserted into the middle of the femur and kept in place by cement. The surgeon will then allow the ball to slip into its new socket, thereby giving you a new hip.

All that remains to be done is to stitch the muscles and skin. A dressing is then placed over the original incision and the operation is completed.

What happens after the operation?

Before the operation your surgeon will have emphasized to you the importance of the post-operative period, for it is then that you will have to play your part in the proceedings to ensure a successful outcome.

Surgeons have differing post-operative routines, but normally you will be in bed for the first 48 hours following your operation. During this period you will be visited by the physiotherapist, who will encourage you to move your legs. You must do this for two reasons. First, to prevent the possibility of blood clots forming in the veins and, second, as the initial phase in rebuilding the strength in the muscles surrounding your hip, so that when you begin to bear weight your hip will be strong enough to take the strain.

Following this initial stay in bed, you will gradually be mobilized under the strict supervision of the physiotherapists. They will gradually encourage you to allow increasing weight-bearing on your hip, though always with supports such as parallel bars, crutches and walkers. Nowadays, increasing use is being made of hydrotherapy pools to encourage non-weight-bearing mobilization of post-operative hips.

When, eventually, discharge is decided upon, you will be allowed home, although this will be with the proviso that over the next four to six weeks, you should consider yourself very much in a convalescence period and you will be advised exactly what you may and may not do.

During this convalescence period you will attend the out-patients' department to see your consultant as well as the physiotherapy department, where the physiotherapists will assess and advise upon further exercises to encourage the strengthening of your hip muscles.

If all goes well, after about 12 weeks you should be able to begin to go about your normal activities, though if you are uncertain as to how much you should be doing you should ask your surgeon or physiotherapist for advice.

What arthritic problems can occur in my knees?

Having gone into hip replacement in some detail, I should now like to briefly answer some of your questions on other surgical procedures that can help in both rheumatoid arthritis and osteoarthritis.

One of the areas where the greatest advances have recently been made is in the surgical treatment of arthritis of the knee. One of the main problems that can arise in arthritis of the knees is the fact that due to the chronic pain that can be present, the patient finds it difficult to bear weight and as a consequence the major muscle mass that gives stability to the knee, known as the quadriceps muscle, becomes weakened, thereby making an already unstable and painful joint even more unstable.

Another problem with rheumatoid arthritis of the knee is that the most comfort that can be gained is to have the knee slightly bent. But doing this can leave the knee in a fixed position. When in bed never use a pillow to support your knees in a bent position. This can lead to permanent flexion contracture deformity – in other words, your knees will remain permanently bent. To prevent this, gentle passive exercises are advised – such as extending the knee from time to time while sitting down.

One of the problems with arthritic knee joints is getting up from chairs and I think you may find the following tips helpful. Get yourself as far forwards in the chair as possible and then place your palms as near to your thighs as possible. Then, gently lean forwards, pushing up with your hands. As you will realize, this will have the effect of both lifting you from the chair and also straightening your knees, while putting less than normal stress upon your knee joints. While you are doing all this, try and keep your knees as far apart as possible.

At what stage would my surgeon consider operating on my arthritic knees?

One of the major considerations will be the amount of pain that you are experiencing. If this really has reached the stage where you feel happier sitting down all the time and you find yourself confined to a single chair, then this would weigh heavily with your surgeon's decision to operate.

He will also be guided by the amount of joint irregularity that he can assess from your X-rays. Finally, if physiotherapy combined with drugs and injections into the joint are all failing to help, he will almost certainly advise a knee replacement operation in which an artificial joint will be inserted to take the place of your functionless knee.

Following your operation, it is particularly important that you appreciate the need for physiotherapy and rehabilitation. Initially you will not be allowed to bear weight on your knee, and your walking will be assisted by various forms of support such as crutches or modified walking frames.

During the immediate post-operative period, in hospital, not only will your walking receive much attention but so also will building the strength in the muscles surrounding the knee joint, because it is the support of these muscles that will give the joint its long-term stability. After about two weeks' intensive therapy you will probably be ready for discharge although for about the next two months you will need the support of crutches.

Do not be worried if things seem to be progressing slowly, for it can take anything up to six months before the new joint and its surrounding muscles have settled into harmonious place.

What surgical operations can be used to help arthritis of the wrist and hand?

There are a great variety of operations that can be done in both rheumatoid arthritis and osteoarthritis of the wrist and hand. Most involve treatment to the tendons and their sheaths that are so prone to damage by the arthritic process, although the replacement of an arthritic wrist with an artificial joint is becoming a more common operation.

There is another problem that is not in itself arthritic but that is commonly encountered in arthritis in this area. This is carpal tunnel syndrome (see p.18).

What other surgical solutions are there to arthritic problems in the hand?

One of the main problems of rheumatoid arthritis of the hand is the involvement of the tendons – the direct extensions of the muscles that allow for many of the delicate hand movements. In order to move easily, these tendons are enclosed within a sheath, lined by synovial membrane, which, you will recall, lines the inner aspect of the knee joint. It is the swelling and inflammation of this synovial membrane that is at the basis of rheumatoid arthritis and, if it occurs around the tendons of the hand, can cause restricted and painful movements of the fingers.

One way in which this problem can be solved is by the actual removal, or excision, of these inflamed synovial sheaths, the operation being technically called synovectomy.

Sometimes, the synovial membrane can become so intrusive and inflamed that it may actually cause the tendons to weaken, and on occasion they can rupture. In such cases, an operation to repair the tendons concerned is necessitated.

In advanced cases of hand deformity, where the tendons have become very contracted and are no longer able to allow the hand to carry out delicate movements, a variety of operations can be carried out that involve transferring some of the tendons from one part of the hand to another where their actions are better employed.

Although these tendon transplant procedures cannot restore the hand's original function, they can, in certain patients, return useful function to a previously malfunctioning hand.

Can surgery help backache caused by arthritis?

Surgery certainly has a place in the treatment of back problems that give intractable pain but when that pain is due to either rheumatoid arthritis or osteoarthritis its applications are very limited.

You may recall that earlier (p.33) I discussed the structure of the vertebral column. Although at first sight the spinal column appears to be fairly rigid in nature, it is, in fact, made up of a series of bones, called vertebrae, which sit upon each other, rather like a stack of single bricks. Each vertebra is able to move independently with its neighbour both above and below it by means of a series of small but highly refined articular joints which, although they do not permit great movement, allow for the suppleness of the spinal column that is so characteristic of childhood and early adulthood.

Just as this great number of small articulations is so useful to us in order that we may both flex and extend our backs, these joints are prone to both rheumatoid and osteoarthritis. This is not to say, of course, that all back pain is due to either rheumatoid arthritis or osteoarthritis. Indeed, back problems – especially when they involve the lower back – are an area of diagnosis that presents difficulties to almost every doctor. This problem mainly arises because in and around the spinal column there are not only a large number of small joints that allow the vertebrae to articulate but, between the joints are discs, known as intervertebral discs, which prevent the vertebrae from grating upon each other. If, in some way or another, these discs become displaced or lose their inherent elasticity, this leads to a relative compression of the spinal column, which can result in entrapment of nerves that run through holes in the spinal column. This process can, as a consequence, give rise to much pain and is known as 'slipped disc'.

But it is not only these factors that can give rise to back pain. The whole spinal column is surrounded by a number of inter-locking muscles and ligaments, strains of which give rise to pain and instability of the spinal column.

So, as I am sure that you can now see, the back and vertebral column is far from being the inert structure that at first sight it seems to be. Rather, it is a multiplicity of muscles, ligaments, joints, discs and nerves that are designed to work in the closest harmony. It takes only one element of this orchestra to play out of tune for the whole orchestra to falter. It is these subtle changes in the nature of the back's anatomy, which can also have carry-over effects, that make the elucidation of such problems so difficult. And so makes surgery for the particular problem of arthritis of these small joints so unsatisfactory.

Can sciatica caused by arthritis of the spine be treated by surgery?

Sciatica is a commonly misunderstood term. In fact, it has a very specific meaning. When the sciatic nerve – the largest nerve that travels to the legs – emerges from between the two lower vertebrae that make up the lumbar spinal column, it can find itself trapped by either a slipped disc or an arthritic outgrowth called an osteophyte. When this occurs, the patient normally complains of a pain beginning in the buttock and running down the leg, and exacerbated by movement of the spinal column or of the affected leg. In some cases surgery to remove the prolapsed disc or the protruding osteophyte is advised.

Is there anything that I can do to help my back pain?

There are a number of things that you can do in general terms to look after your back.

I am sure that many of you will remember that when you went to tea at Grandma's you were probably placed in a particularly uncomfortable chair with a even more uncomfortable straight back to it. You almost certainly found that this hard, straight back had the effect of barely allowing you to sit upon the chair because Grandma's paramount concern was the fact that without good posture, your back might, in later years, suffer the most horrendous deformities. And, of course, she was right.

So, one thing that we can all do to help our backs is to try as much as possible to use sensible chairs. Chairs that leave our backs with good support and posture.

But, if Grandma would have been horrified by our modern seating apparatus, just think what her thoughts would have been had she seen some of the beds that we use. Considering the amount of time that we spend in bed during our lifetime, it is not surprising that so many of us have back problems. Just think how much time our backs lie, relatively unsupported, in those lovely, deep sagging sumptuous beds that do our spinal columns no good at all.

If you have a back problem, it is probably a good, long-term idea to buy a bed and mattress that give your back decent support. Don't go overboard and get something distinctly uncomfortable, but try and reach a happy medium: comfort with support.

And now to the subject of lifting weights which, I am convinced, is the root cause of may people's back problems. The cardinal rule is this: never ever, when lifting any sort of weight, do so with the knees straight and the back bent. When you are lifting any sort of weight, keep the back as straight as possible and lower yourself to pick up the load by bending your knees. Your knee joints are immensely strong whereas your vertebral joints, while strong, have nothing like the weight-bearing properties of your knee joints. Let your knee joints and not your vertebral joints take the strain, therefore.

Can corsets be of any help in arthritis of the spine?

Corsets can be of great help if used correctly and under medical supervision. It is important to be aware of the place that they occupy in the therapy of back problems for there are some people with low back problems who, without medical advice, buy themselves a corset and can, in fact, do themselves rather more harm than good. If you are thinking of getting a corset to help you with your back problem, do seek professional advice before doing so.

In the acute phase of a painful low back, lumbar corsets do not probably have a very useful role. During this acutely painful period, the patient is normally receiving specific treatment such as traction or bedrest on a suitably hard surface, as well as a range of pain-killing and anti-inflammatory tablets. Once this acute stage is over, however, the lumbar corset can be of great help.

It is important to realize that the function of such a corset is not to immobilize the spine but, rather, to restrict it from making unnatural and awkward movements which may aggravate the situation and give rise, once more, to the acutely painful back.

However, a word of warning. Your back problems will *not* be solved simply by wearing a lumbar corset. Even though the corset is being worn you must adopt a proper posture and protect your back at all times – especially when lifting. It is also important that you continue your exercises, and this is something the lumbar corset will not do for you.

When you have taken your corset off and are in bed, do not forget that your back is now lacking support, and do go to sensible lengths to ensure that the mattress and the bed are continuing to support your lumbar spine.

Is neck pain always due to arthritis?

The simple answer to this question is, no. Cervical pain – otherwise called neck pain – can be due to rheumatoid arthritis as well as osteoarthritis.

One of the problems in diagnosing neck pain is the fact that sometimes the pain is due to spasm of the muscles that surround the neck, a secondary reaction to an initiating cause. Often, this initiating cause cannot be pin-pointed with total accuracy, though the muscle spasm itself may be amenable to a number of local treatments.

But, let us return for a moment to the causes of neck pain. Apart from rheumatoid arthritis and osteoarthritis, there are other conditions that can give rise to neck pain.

One of these is the presence of osteophytes – small bony protuberances that can grow out from the cervical bones. Osteophytes are part of the osteoarthritic ageing process of the cervical spine. They can either impinge upon the large number of nerves in the region, thus disturbing neck movements, or grate and dig into the surrounding neck muscles, giving rise to painful spasm.

Another, not infrequent cause of neck pain – also due to a structure impinging on local nerves and muscles – is the protrusion of one of the discs between the cervical vertebrae, known as a cervical slipped disc. These problems can be compounded by secondary effects, as a result of recent or old injury as well as, rarely, infections and cancers.

Finally, there is a group of patients who experience pain but in whom no physical abnormalities can be found. In some of these cases there is undoubtedly a psychological aspect to the problem. But it is very wrong to automatically label neck pain as psychological until all aspects of the problem have been taken into account. For instance, a patient may mention that he is undergoing great stress at work, and the unwary doctor may immediately latch on to this statement, putting the neck pain down to stress at work. If questioned more closely, however, it is quite possible that working conditions such as having to spend long hours looking at a computer may have given rise to abnormal neck posture. But although the work is stressful, it is actually the adverse physical working conditions that are causing the problem.

Can cervical collars help with arthritis of the neck?

Cervical collars can be of great help in relieving pain that arises either from the cervical spine or the soft tissues surrounding the spine. But it is also important to understand that, in some cases, a cervical collar can cause more problems than it solves, because of the wide-ranging nature of the causes of cervical pain. True, both osteoarthritis and rheumatoid arthritis can be causes of such pain but there are also others, including spasm in the muscles that surround the cord and the upper shoulders. Thus, simply giving a cervical support for neck pain may not always be the answer.

One of the conditions where a cervical collar *is* of use, however, is in osteoarthritis of the cervical column. In this condition, quite apart from the pain that is generated by the specific areas of osteoarthritis that form upon the joints of the cervical column, there is also the secondary effect of spasm of the muscles that are attached, at their upper ends, to the cervical vertebrae and, at their lower ends, to the shoulder blades. Under these circumstances, as well as locally applied heat, together with exercises supervised by the physiotherapist, a cervical collar is often prescribed.

However, do not suppose that the purpose of this collar is to support the neck. This is a common assumption that is not true. The purpose of the cervical collar is to cause the neck to be slightly bent forwards, to be flexed. The effect of this is to lessen the strain on the muscles surrounding the cervical column, the spasm in which can give rise to so much of the pain as a secondary effect of the cervical osteoarthritis.

Although cervical collars can give great comfort, it is important to remember that any muscle group in the body, if it is not used, becomes weak. Therefore, it is important to keep these muscle groups active and working. Do not become too reliant upon your cervical collar. Take it off for a certain amount of time each day, as your physiotherapist advises, to allow the muscles of the neck to exercise themselves.

At night time it is usually recommended that the cervical collar be taken off. But in such cases it is important that all the good work done during the day is not wasted during the sleeping hours. A good compromise is a cervical pillow, which can, in a limited way, fulfil the same functions during sleep that the cevical collar fulfils during waking hours.

How can the depression that inevitably comes with arthritis be treated and coped with?

When doctors talk of depression they tend to divide the causes into two main areas. The first, known as endogenous depression, arises from within and appears on the surface, to have no justifiable cause. It is assumed that the causes of this type of depression arise from specific, but as yet unknown, chemical defects in those cells of the brain that are responsible for mood.

But, by far and away the largest group of patients who suffer from depression are those who quite obviously have something to be depressed about. And it is into this group that arthritic patients who become depressed tend to fall. It is completely understandable that a formerly healthy person who finds himself quite unexpectedly having to cope with an arthritic problem should react in this manner.

Apart from the direct problem of having to come to terms with an illness, indirect problems may arise which, in themselves can cause depression. For example, an employer may decide that the arthritic patient is a burden rather than a help (in the vast majority of cases this is quite patently untrue, even though the arthritic sufferer may have to take time off work).

Also, it is sometimes difficult for some of the members of the arthritic sufferer's family – especially a spouse – to come to terms with the fact that a formerly healthy member of the family now needs a lot of attention.

Loss of independence is a further problem that has to be accepted in some cases. There are many aspects of their former lives that patients can no longer enjoy, and indeed, I am always struck by the fact that there does not appear to be more depressive illness in arthritic sufferers than is normally found.

There are countless reasons for feeling unhappy and depressed with having to cope with arthritis and so it is important that the psychological aspects of arthritis are fully faced. The worst thing that you can do is to bottle it all up. If you are feeling depressed, unhappy, sad, anxious, talk about it, and talk through it. This must be the initial step towards coping with the problem. Once you start talking about things you will find that this, in itself, can lighten the psychological burden.

There are a number of reasons why it is important for you to talk about your depressive problems. First – and I know that this may appear obvious – if you don't start to talk about your problem, if you don't confide in somebody, then the problem that you are bottling up will only get worse. Second, one of the main reasons for the failure of treatment is a lack of frank understanding and co-operation between doctor and patient which may include a denial of depression.

If you feel depressed, you will invariably lack motivation. And it is motivation, above all else, that is absolutely essential when undergoing any form of long-term therapy, whether it involves simply taking tablets or more elaborate forms of treatment such as having to undertake a series of particular exercises that may be boring, time-consuming and, on occasions, painful. This may often also be combined with an uncomfortable and long journey in either car or ambulance to your local physiotherapy department.

Depression can make all these tasks all the more harder. Which is why it is so important to eliminate depression, because treatment, and especially long-term treatment, is such an important part of controlling the disease.

In recent years many arthritic sufferers' groups have sprung up, all over the country. I would strongly recommend that you join one of these, if you have not already done so, for shared experience can be extremely helpful.

If you find that you are unable to join one of these local groups please look towards the end of this book where you will find a number of useful addresses of associations which are particularly helpful, in this respect (p.146).

But this still leaves the problems of having to come to terms with accepting that I have arthritis. How can this problem be overcome?

In this increasingly complex world, all of us – including those of us who are lucky enough not to suffer from any major disease – realize that we have to cope with problems of a psychological nature that are both a part of ourselves and also arise from the stresses and strains of the society in which we live.

At times, such psychological problems can appear almost too much to bear. Understandably, many sufferers of rheumatic diseases ask, 'Why me? I've enough to cope with, as it is. Why, with all the problems and stresses of the society within which I live do I have to live with this additional problem, this wretched arthritic condition?' And certainly, I find this a morally impossible question to grapple with. Why should some people be struck down with what is, in some cases, a crippling disease and have to cope with it, together with all the other problems that follow in its wake, as well as all the normal problems of our complex society?

I frankly find it philosophically impossible to produce an answer to this question, which is why I feel that it is important that the concept of acceptance of disease be faced. Once this is faced, and conquered, other psycho-social problems can themselves be faced more easily and readily.

Coming to terms with the disease, especially arthritic in nature, coming to accept all the problems that it throws up, is not a thing that most people find easy. When a relative or a friend, or even just a passing acquaintance, realizes that you suffer with arthritis it is more often the immediacy of the physical disability that grips their attention and, not being sufferers themselves, they find it difficult to see past this and to appreciate the other, rather more subtle, problems that the disease can present.

For instance, somebody who has hitherto been a particularly independent person, even though they may not be suffering from a severe form of arthritis, may find that even a certain amount of restriction of their independence means a great loss to them, not only in physical terms, but also in psychological terms, in the knowledge that they can no longer do what they had always assumed they would have no trouble in doing. This very real demonstration of loss of physical ability can often give rise to a loss of inner self-confidence which can, in some cases, be far more devastating than the disease itself.

In a disease with such striking elements of subjective qualities, it is often difficult to assess the progressive nature of the disease and the effect that the treatment is having upon that progression when these overlying psychological factors form a part of the overall equation.

But, there is one thing that can quite definitely be stated and that is that psychological factors have no part in the cause of either rheumatoid arthritis or osteoarthritis, even though, as I have just explained, it is quite possible that arthritis and its psychological consequences can bring to the surface personality traits such as anxiety or depression that might not otherwise have been suspected.

It has also been suggested that stress can cause an acute exacerbation of arthritis but there is no real hard-and-fast evidence to support this, though it is certainly true that in highly stressful situations, symptoms of rheumatoid arthritis can, indeed, be exacerbated.

One of the goals to aim for, strange though it may seem at first sight, is some sort of appreciation and acceptance that the disease is present and that it is going to cause certain limitations to your future lifestyle.

I do not make this suggestion glibly. It is based upon a well-known psychological route that wends its way through most chronic illnesses. Initially, when the diagnosis is first made, there is inevitably a period of time during which, even in the face of incontrovertible medical evidence, the patient says to himself 'it can't be me'. Then, once he realizes that he has the disease, there is a period during which a certain amount of anger and self-pity can occur, and this is more than understandable. A depressive phase sometimes follows, during which things can look very black and there appears to be no light at the end of the tunnel. Then, gradually, once this phase is worked through, there appears, on the horizon, an acceptance of the problem and of its consequences. Not a passive acceptance, not a laying-down of resistance, but, rather, a new starting-point. An acceptance that a disease is present but, at the same time, with a realization that there is a very definite future, filled with hope. Once this stage has been reached, coping with the disease itself is invariably altogether a much easier proposition.

What about problems with sexual activity. Who can I turn to and what do I ask about?

This is a very touchy subject, even in these so-called liberated times. In general terms, it is probably easier to talk about your sexual problem with somebody of the same sex in your theraupeutic team. Once the ice is broken, you will often find it much easier to talk openly about the problem.

Nowadays, health professionals are well aware of the particular problems in this area experienced by people with arthritis, and you will undoubtedly, at some stage of your assessment, have this question tactfully brought up, so that, if you wish to discuss it further, you will be able so to do. If you feel unable to talk about it, however, you will not be pressed to do so.

What is the importance of co-operation between doctor and patient?

There are inevitably two aspects to this question. On the one hand there is the doctor who has explained to the arthritic patient how to take the prescribed treatment, how to apply splints, if these are required, the amount of rest to be taken and specific instructions as to how much exercise should be taken. Picture, then, this same doctor, who, having given these instructions, sees, over a series of successive visits, that his patient seems to be getting worse, rather than better. Imagine also what goes through his mind when he eventually learns that the reason for the steady decline in his patient's condition is due to the fact that the tablets are sometimes not being taken by the patient, or, the splints are not being applied, or the exercises are being done only intermittently.

But what about the doctor's role, in all this? I hear you say. And, of course, you're quite right. This is the other aspect to the question. It is undeniably true that it is often the doctor's inability to communicate to the patient what exactly is required of him that can lead to this breakdown in communication and understanding. In other words, patient and doctor must be frank with each other. If a doctor sees that his treatment is not working, he must first ask himself if he has explained fully and precisely what it is that he expects of his patient as regards the taking of treatment. If so satisfied, he must then, at the risk of offending his patient, enquire frankly whether he or she is carrying out the treatment programme.

If, on the other hand, you as the patient, do not understand what your doctor has said to you, you must ask for a clarification of the instructions. I know that this is easier said than done, for we live in an imperfect world where appointments are all too short both from doctor's and patient's point of view. The doctor knows that he has only a certain limited amount of time in which to not only make the diagnosis but also to decide upon treatment. To be honest, it is often the fault of the doctor that he spends far too little time in, firstly, explaining the nature of the disease and, secondly, explaining how the treatments that he is prescribing should be taken for best effect.

If you have not fully understood what your doctor has said to you, if you feel that somehow there is some pressure on you during the consultation, in that your doctor appears to be in a hurry, don't worry. Go away, think about what he has said to you and write down on a piece of paper the questions that have arisen in your mind. Then, when you have a clear idea of the various points that you would like to have elucidated, make a further appointment with your doctor. Tell him that you have not come for a further examination or indeed a repeat prescription for the tablets that he has given you, but that there are certain points that you would like elaborated. Don't worry. He certainly won't feel that you're wasting his time. In the long run he knows that you will be saving it. Every doctor knows that unless the disease process and its treatment is fully explained the chances of a patient taking the prescribed treatment is probably less that 50 per cent.

It is in everybody's interests, therefore, for both doctor and patient to be frank with each other, with each being absolutely sure that the other is quite clear as to what is expected of them. This simple matter of good communication can go a long way to resolving one of the main causes of disappointments in treatments either because the doctor has not taken time enough to explain in detail to his patient, what the problem is and how he proposes to solve it, or on the other hand, the patient is sometimes reluctant to continue with treatment in which he has little or no confidence in, because of uncertainty as to what the actually problem is.

What part will understanding the principles of my therapy have to play in the nature of my condition?

In no other disease is patient education more important than in arthritis. I do feel, however, that not only in the field of arthritis but in medicine generally it is very important to explain to patients the basic principles underlying their disease and the treatment that they are being given for that disease.

A typical example is exercise and arthritis, which I have already touched upon. Gone are the days when a patient is just simply told what to do. We are now living in an era of medicine when, for instance, not only is the purpose of exercise explained but also the reasons why, say, too much exercise in certain circumstances, or, too little exercise in others, can be harmful. It is no longer a question of simply giving the instruction, 'Do these specific exercises for that specific amount of time.'

Similarly, joint protection is of prime importance, so no longer should we, as doctors, simply tell the patient, 'Protect that joint with this splint,' but, rather, explain to him what will happen if the joint is not adequately protected. In my experience, if patients understand *why* they are receiving a certain treatment, they will be far more enthusiastic in carrying that treatment out.

Another good example of proper explanation is the question of diets. Because of the nature of arthritis – in that it is a disease that waxes and wanes – it is terribly easy to make a claim for one particular diet, or the exclusion of certain foodstuffs because, inevitably, if the diet is long enough, at some stage there will be an improvement in the overall condition that would probably have occurred anyway, without the diet. Nevertheless, it is very wrong, when a patient asks his doctor if a certain diet is worthwhile trying, for that doctor to dismiss the idea completely out of hand. For, although the doctor may know, in his heart of hearts, that the patient is wasting his time by keeping to a specific diet, the patient will feel, quite naturally, antagonistic towards the doctor, because the quick dismissal will have induced in his mind the idea that his doctor thinks he is a crank.

To a large extent, this is the doctor's fault, for he really should sit down and explain, why, in the main, outlandish diets are of no help whatsoever. In this way, by explaining things to patients and educating them, understanding and co-operation is greatly enhanced. But, remember, your doctor can only explain if you ask questions. Don't be afraid to ask these questions, for he will be only too glad to answer them.

But education is not solely restricted to the patient. As I have said, the arthritis sufferer is normally a part of a family or some other form of social grouping. In this case, not only is explanation to the patient of supreme importance, but also an education of the social group within which that patient is living. If, for instance, the family is given an understanding of the arthritic process together with a practical explanation of the treatment many positive results may follow. The patient will feel more settled in his mind in the knowledge that his social grouping has been made more aware by an independent person of his problem and the social grouping itself, with an understanding of the problem, will feel relieved that it is more able to help the arthritic sufferer. A side-effect of this is that the social group can give positive encouragement to the arthritic sufferer during those very natural periods of depression when the disease appears to be insurmountable.

Alternative Therapies

Can acupuncture therapy help my arthritis?

Acupunture is a form of therapy that in the past has been considered to be outside orthodox medical treatment. It is politely termed an 'alternative' therapy to what is considered to be the traditional approach to the treatment of arthritis as practised by the medical establishment.

Of late, however, acupuncture has been drawing more than just a passing interest from both patients and physicians, because there are accumulating reports that, in certain circumstances, it has a positive place in the treatment of arthritis.

What is acupuncture?

There are a number of different forms of acupuncture therapy but each specific approach works on the basis that there are small, specific areas, either on or just beneath the skin, that are neurologically connected with anatomical structures within the body. These specific points are connected by 12 lines, or meridians, that can be traced on the body's skin.

When specific anatomical structures become diseased their acupunture points become accentuated. This accentuation is recognized and then mapped out by the acupuncturist. By mapping out points which, for instance, appear to be tender, a diagnosis may then be made.

Therapy is given by stimulating these acupuncture points, either by simple pressure or by inserting fine needles into the skin at the sites of these points. Stimulation is then given by simple rotation of the needle or by more sophisticated methods of electrical stimulation.

How does acupuncture therapy work?

Currently, some scientists believe that by stimulating acupuncture points, natural chemicals within the substance of the brain, called endorphins, are released. It is thought that endorphins are naturally occurring pain relieving chemicals and so cause the relief of painful arthritis in the best physiological way possible. Whether or not this will turn out to be the case, only time will tell.

One interesting point about acupuncture is that very few acupuncturists will claim that it can reverse the physical and pathological damage that arthritis does to the joints. For instance, an arthritic hip cannot be returned to its non-arthritic state by acupuncture. What the acupuncturist will claim, however, is that the pain and problems associated with the arthritic hip can be dissipated by his therapy.

Does acupuncture therapy work and, if so, how?

With any treatment, whether orthodox or 'alternative', there are always problems in accurately assessing whether it is effective or not. In certain circumstances, it can be clearly shown that the orthodox method is the most effective. A typical example is appendicitis, where by taking out the inflamed appendix the patient can be completely cured. In the case of a chronic and intermittently remitting disease, such as arthritis, however, the assessment is far less clear-cut. It is well known that arthritis waxes and wanes. If treatment is given during an exacerbation of the arthritis, it is unclear, when relief comes, whether or not the treatment has produced the desired effect or whether the improvement in the patient's wellbeing has come about as a natural remission in the disease process.

So how can I know if the acupuncture is working?

Probably by listening to those who have received acupuncture. It must be admitted that the majority of people suffering with arthritis who have undergone acupuncture therapy admit to an improvement of their arthritic condition, albeit temporarily.

Should I take up acupuncture therapy, then?

If you have found that orthodox therapy has not brought you the relief that you had hoped for, go and discuss acupuncture with your doctor. He may not feel that acupuncture is going to help you but even if this is the case, it is still important that he realizes both the frustration you feel with your present treatment and your desire to try an 'alternative' approach. Whatever his reaction, it is very important that you tell him if you *do* decide to take up acupuncture, because if he doesn't realize that you are having this treatment he may well feel, when you do not return to him for some time that it is his therapy that is working rather than the acupuncture.

If you do try acupuncture therapy, be sure to go to an acupuncturist who is registered with an authorized body or organisation. Finally, don't be too disappointed if it does not give the permanent relief that is often claimed by those who practise this art.

What role does osteopathy have in the treatment of arthritis?

This is an area of medicine that is always difficult to evaluate. Before doctors are satisfied with a particular treatment, they like to see the scientific evidence, in black and white. Unfortunately, osteopathy does not lend itself to precise scientific measurement of this sort. The patient may feel better after his back has been manipulated, but for how long? In the long run, for instance, is it going to make his back problem worse? Or, would his back problem have got worse, anyway? Such are the problems of assessing the merits of manipulative osteopathy.

Is it advisable to seek help from an osteopath?

If the osteopath you consult claims that he can cure your arthritis steer clear of that sort of promise. Reputable osteopaths, including doctors who specialize in osteopathy, will never claim that they can cure arthritis. What the genuine osteopath can often do, by manipulation of particular joints, to bring considerable symptomatic relief, especially to intractable back problems.

If you are interested in trying osteopathy, speak to your doctor. He will probably be able to recommend someone to you. But, before you go to an osteopath make sure that there is nothing seriously wrong with your back – you will remember that earlier I mentioned various diseases of the back and elsewhere in the body that can cause back pain problems which can all too easily be put down to arthritis of the spine.

Can homeopathy be of any use in treating arthritis?

Every day millions of people worldwide are treated by homeopathy. It is a therapy that is available on the National Health Service. The principle upon which homeopathy is based is that those substances that create signs and symptoms in healthy individuals can be used to combat diseases which produce similar clinical pictures. The more dilute these substances are the more efficacious they are said to be.

Clearly, the treatment of advanced osteoarthritis of the hip will not be achieved by homeopathic remedies. But in the earlier stages of rheumatoid arthritis and osteoarthritis there appears to be some evidence to suggest that the progression of these diseases can be beneficially altered by certain homeopathic remedies.

However, before embarking on such a line of therapy do discuss the matter fully with your own doctor. Certainly homeopathy is, in the main, safe – something which, sadly, cannot be said of many of our more modern medications for the treatment of arthritis.

What is transcutaneous electrical nerve stimulation?

This form of pain relief in arthritis is becoming more widely available and offers instant and real results. It entails placing two electrodes at specific sites in areas of arthritic pain. The siting of these electrodes is crucially important and is normally a question of trial and error. A small, direct current is then passed between the two electrodes giving a tingling sensation.

Obviously, the pain relief will be different in certain individuals, but in general terms, this therapy does seem to offer a safe and effective method of treating some of the pain caused by arthritis.

Adapting Your Lifestyle

How can I adapt my lifestyle to my arthritic condition?

I think that one of the most crucial points in deciding how best to adapt to a lifestyle that has to take account of arthritis is to appreciate that a balance must be found between, on the one hand, considering how best to protect the affected joints while, at the same time, not having to be restricted to a sedentary lifestyle that takes much of the enjoyment out of day-to-day living.

First, it is a fact of the disease process that during each day you will require more rest than you will have been used to – both for your complete body and for the affected joints. However, at this stage I must re-emphasize that both periods of general rest and also the rest of specific joints will differ from one individual to another so you must be guided by the medical advice that you are given that takes account of your particular problem. In many cases, for example, it is inadvisable to stay in bed for long periods, for although, at the time, such rest may give great comfort and relief, it can allow the muscles surrounding the joint to develop contractures and, in some cases, to become subsequently weakened. There will inevitably be times, however, when the problem will flare up and, during these episodes, more than usual bed rest is advisable.

But with rheumatoid arthritis, there is another factor that is sometimes overlooked. This is something that is still not fully explained on scientific grounds, but it is well known that the body can generally feel tired and exhausted during a flare-up of one or more joints. It is, therefore, important to adapt your daily routine to take account of those periods when not only the joints flare up but also when you feel tired and fatigued.

This general tiredness and fatigue must also be taken into

account when deciding upon daily activities. Even when resting in bed, it is important to remember that certain joints, even though you may feel that they are being adequately rested, may require a certain amount of splinting for their protection, and simple adaptation to this helpful form of mechanical treatment is often necessary.

On the other hand, when these symptoms appear to have improved, don't feel that now is the time to do all those jobs that you could not get around to doing while you were having to take enforced bed rest because excessive activity can in itself cause a flare-up of the rheumatic process. Be sensible. Do what you feel that you can manage without putting undue stress upon your body and your joints.

Another important point to remember when adapting your lifestyle to your condition is that you will have to allow time for the specific exercises that you will have been prescribed by either your doctor or your physiotherapist and find time to fit these into your daily routine. Remember that, even though you may think that you are exercising while, say, you are doing housework, it is possible that such exercise is not quite what the doctor ordered for that specific joint.

As well as the physical aspects of your daily routine you must also set aside time for prescribed exercise.

Here are some practical points to help you to adapt your lifestyle to your condition.

First, before you do anything, decide what is the easiest way of going about it. Try and see how you can best conserve your energy whilst performing the task. Don't charge in and then halfway through the job, realize that you have bitten off more than you can chew. One of the most important things to think about is the time that you are going to allow yourself, not only for doing and completing the specific task but also the time that you must allow for your body and joints to completely recover, once the task is completed.

In other words, don't set yourself impossible goals. If anything, err on the side of doing too little rather than too much. We all know what is possible and what is impossible. Don't try the impossible and then become depressed with the realization that you cannot complete your goal.

Let's take a practical example, Imagine that you've decided to cook a slap-up meal. You have decided what you are going to cook, so obviously you're going to have to go out and buy the ingredients. If you can get somebody to go out and to do the shopping for you, all well and good. But what if you can't and the meal's going to be a surprise, and you want to do the shopping yourself? Think about it. Even if you didn't have arthritis, what would you do? You'd start by making out a list. But, why not be a little bit more specific? With your list in front of you, decide from which shops you're going to buy the various items and see if it is possible to save yourself going to all the shops listed by combining as many purchases as possible in as few shops, as possible.

This brings me to another point. Before you get to each individual shop, you will almost certainly have been there before. Why not plan out the route that you're going to take, around the shop, bearing energy-saving in mind?

So now your shopping's done. You have your bits and pieces and you are back in your kitchen. Are you organized in your kitchen? There are many books and pamphlets, some extremely well illustrated, as to how best to organize your kitchen for such situations but, in the main, this sort of organization is simply common sense.

Here are some basic ideas that can help you.

Think of the common, everyday things that are always in use and have these on the work surfaces, ready to hand. Don't keep them in the deep recesses of your cupboards where you've got to constantly be taking them in and out. Think about washing up, and the utensils that you are going to be frequently using and always keep these in or near the sink.

The same goes for your cooker and your cooking utensils – keep them as near the cooker as possible. For instance, if you have oven mittens for handling hot dishes keep these near the stove and not tucked away in some obscure drawer, on the other side of the kitchen.

Most important of all, when cooking the meal, try and sit down as much as possible.

This buying and preparing a meal, although I have skipped lightly over it, really serves to emphasize the prime lesson of thinking through an activity before you embark upon it. You will frequently surprise yourself as you come to realize how much energy can be unnecessarily wasted if your task has not been thoroughly thought through.

So, a part of adapting your lifestyle to your rheumatic condition is very much a question of planning. Thinking through the various tasks that you have to perform on a daily basis and, before performing them, deciding how best, on theoretical grounds, you can approach the variety of problems that these tasks throw up. By doing this you will save yourself expending and wasting unnecessary energy.

How can I adapt my lifestyle to cope with fatigue?

First, take a good look at your general day-to-day activities. I'm sure that when you do this you will immediately find ways of cutting down on the energy needed to perform many of your routine tasks.

Take, for instance, making a bed. Make one side completely, then do the same with the other side rather than going backwards and forwards and expending unnecessary energy.

Another important factor is training yourself to sense when you are about to become fatigued and to take a rest before you become too tired. Don't overdo things, and do as much of your work as possible sitting down. The following point may seem a little selfish but I assure you that it is not. Try and encourage those around you to do as much for themselves, as possible. Families, especially, must appreciate that they will have to do more than they used to do in and around the home, now that you can't do so much. There are more specific points you can remember, too. As far as clothes are concerned, select those that will give you the least trouble in putting them on and taking them off.

Think about where you are going to put things in your house, bearing easy accessibility in mind.

Finally, one tip that I think is very useful is to have a diary or a wall planner and put down everything that you expect to be doing over, for instance, the next two weeks. And I mean everything. *Not* just social events. Once you have done this, you will realize you are duplicating many tasks. A definite written plan also has the advantage of ensuring that you give yourself enough time to rest.

Make planning an essential part of your life. It may seem rather a lot of work at first, but will be worth it in the long run.

Can mechanical aids help in normal daily tasks?

Yes, there are a vast number of implements on the market, that have been designed to help the arthritis sufferer. Some are excellent, others are just expensive toys. Some are also far too expensive for what they are. Others may be less expensive but may not stand the test of time.

It is therefore important to assess, either on your own, or with the help of such people as doctors, physiotherapists and occupational therapists just what exactly you need for your particular tasks. It is tempting to be offered some flashy-looking gadget for which you can pay a small fortune, but which you may find that you hardly ever use. So, in much the same way as you should plan out your daily living, to take your condition into account, you must apply the same considerations when thinking about what you need in the way of mechanical aids. When choosing these, don't just think about specific tasks. Remember, fatigue is part of the disease process. Look at any mechanical devices, therefore, not only from the viewpoint of their specific functional advantages, but also from that of whether or not, in the long run, they will make the task that you are planning more or less fatiguing. Some devices that I have seen, while making the task itself much easier, have been tiring and fatiguing to use.

Also, do think about the safety aspects of the device. This should be considered from two points of view. First your own personal capabilities. Some of us are more mechanically minded than others. If you fall into the latter category, be realistic. Be frank with yourself. Can you be completely confident? Can you be sure that you will be able to cope with the mechanics of the apparatus? Can you be sure that you will be able to use it in all situations, and that it is not going to be more of an hindrance than a help?

Secondly, look at the apparatus itself, and think about it in your home setting. Might you, unwittingly, cause an accident, in your home with it?

Remember, try and keep mechanical devices as simple and as safe as possible.

It is well recognized that there is a psychological barrier with some patients in accepting mechanical aids. There is both the subconscious fear of loss of independence together with the frequently expressed concern that they will become dependent upon these aids. Be realistic. Think of the tasks that form part of your lifestyle. Then see which of these can be better performed without mechanical aids and which must be performed with aids. There will probably be a grey area, in between and, as far as this is concerned, it is obviously up to the individual to decide whether or not mechanical aids are really a worthwhile investment. You may find that, even with a task that you *think* you will need a mechanical aid for, there may be an alternative way of approaching this without actually buying new apparatus. Finally, remember too that some of these mechanical devices assume that your sight is normal or that many physical activities are unrestricted.

If you decide to buy a mechanical aid, always bear in mind that rheumatoid arthritis is a disease that waxes and wanes, and during those periods when the disease appears to be in remission, set aside as many of your mechanical devices as possible. As long as you feel that you are not overstraining or overstressing yourself, try and carry out your tasks as you used to. Not only will this increase your confidence in yourself, but it will also allow for a limited amount of exercise that will probably be beneficial.

But, be warned. Don't try and do too much. And don't be worried if, halfway through a particular task, you find that you are unable to complete it without the help of your mechanical aid. It is certainly no disgrace to have tried and failed.

One problem that is frequently encountered is that although a mechanical device appears to give the user much more versatility in his particular actions he can, unknowingly and unwittingly, be storing up further problems. This is because some of the devices are necessarily manipulated by joints other than the ones that they are deisgned to help and protect. As a consequence, these joints may themselves be damaged by excessive use.

To conclude, therefore, make sure that although you may be benefiting in the short term, you are not storing up subsequent joint problems for yourself in the long term.

What can I do, architecturally, in my home, to help me get around with my arthritis?

You will find a list of useful addresses on p.146 where you can seek advice on this subject.

Because of the limited scope of this book, I cannot go into specific details with suggestions for every little nook and cranny, both in your house and in your surrounding environment. What I should like to do, however, is mention some aspects of architectural change that will help people with arthritis. Again, I fully realize that I am talking to a broad cross-section of arthritic sufferers, ranging from those who are only mildly affected to those with more severe symptoms.

To all, I would commend the following principles.

Sit down, look around you and think. Think particularly of safety aspects. What can you do in your home to prevent accidents that might occur as a result of your arthritic problem? A common cause of concern and accident, for example, are irregular surfaces – even a small irregularity on a walking surface can cause the arthritic sufferer to trip. Look at your floors, both inside and outside the house, to see if there are any irregularities of the walking surface that can be eliminated. While on the subject of walking surfaces, do also ensure that there are no loose carpet edges sticking up, and, perhaps more importantly, try to get rid of non-fixed carpets and rugs, especially those overlying slippery floors.

Look around you and see where you have steps. Ask yourself whether it is possible to convert these steps into a slope. Also, look at those parts of your house where you find that manoeuvring is difficult, and consider having a railing or a handle to help you manoeuvre yourself more easily or to grab in case of sudden unsteadiness.

Look also at areas that are badly lit – these are frequently areas where accidents can occur. If there is inadequate lighting, have another switch and socket installed.

Thinking further on safety, you must always consider the worst. Although you may feel that you are an extremely careful person, there is always the possibility of fire, in every home. Think, therefore, of where a fire is most likely to occur and then imagine yourself coping with that fire. You might find it helpful to think through the various measures that you could use to put out that fire. Assume that the fire might get out of control. What provision have you made for an emergency exit, from your home? Try and ensure that you have at least two emergency exits from your house even if this means knocking out a window and putting a door in its place.

Talking of doors, what are the knobs on your door like? If they are difficult to use, there are a variety of door knobs designed specifically for arthritis sufferers to make opening and closing doors that much easier.

It is also important that your house, like everyone else's, be secure and this is one area where a lot of useful aids are available. Many security devices such as sophisticated window and door locks tend to be fairly complicated mechanically and for somebody with arthritis – particularly arthritis of the hand – manipulating these security locks is difficult.

However, electronically operated security devices are now coming on to the market. Although these are more expensive, they are easy to use and, in most cases, are more burglar-proof than standard appliances.

What aids are available in the kitchen?

Before describing specific implements, of which there are a legion, I should just like to make some suggestions as to how the general lay-out of a kitchen can be adapted to your best advantage.

Make sure, if needs be, that you have a rail or handle to help you around the kitchen. Also, ensure that the sink you are using is at your optimal height and that the taps on the sink are easy to use. Cooking utensils and irons should be as light as possible and the shelves on which you store them must be at a height that is convenient for you.

As for specifics, we live in an era which, for all of us, has seen an explosion of useful labour-saving devices in the kitchen. As far as your budget will allow, money spent on these implements will be money well spent: ovens and microwaves, built to your specific height requirements, dishwashers and washing machines that are easily accessible; mixers and toasters that are easy to operate.

Apart from these standard fittings, the following are ideas of simple architectural design changes that can be made to your kitchen. (1) Ensure that all work surfaces are built to your particular height requirements. If you do much of your kitchen work in a wheelchair, ensure that the surfaces are high enough for you to allow the wheelchair to manoeuvre beneath them. Have the edge of all work surfaces lined by a rim, half an inch or so in height, to stop articles falling on to the floor. (2) As far as possible, ensure that all drawers pull out and push in as smoothly as possible. This can be achieved by having drawers which slide on ball bearings. (3) Ensure that all handles are large enough to allow you to grip and open them easily. (4) Make sure that all sockets are in easily accessible areas and that you do not have to stretch to plug and unplug. (5) Clothes lines should also be easily accessible. The old-fashioned pulleys that can be raised to the kitchen ceiling are helpful in this respect.

What aids are there to help me with food preparation?

There is a wide range of kitchen aids and gadgets on the market. Think carefully before buying and make sure that what you do buy is really going to be a help and not a hindrance.

You can actually make some devices yourself. A good example is a bread board. All you need do is to knock five nails through the back of your existing board and you will have a spiked area on to which you can place your bread and cut slices without the bread moving.

Mixing bowls with suction bases, mixing jugs, pan holders and recipe book holders can all be modified from existing implements.

Mechanical tin openers, especially the electrical variety, are invaluable while devices for opening tops of jars and bottles will undoubtedly be used by all members of the family.

Special tap extensions are available to make tap turning easier. In the kitchen these are essential and separate turners should be bought for the bathroom and kitchen rather than using one turner for both.

Specially adapted vegetable peelers are very useful, as are specially designed knives with angled handles for cutting meat and bread.

What aids are there for the dining room?

First, a word about moving the prepared food from the kitchen to the dining room. The easiest and safest way to do this is to use a trolley, and you will find that many will double up as an ambulatory aid to walking.

Now, as to the eating aids themselves. A variety of suitable knives, forks and spoons are available. Decide for yourself what suits you best – particularly the shape and size of the handles best suited to your particular hand problem.

Double-handled mugs can greatly facilitate drinking. These can be thermally lined and drinking from them can sometimes more easily be accomplished by using long straws.

Plate surrounds and egg cup holders make stable eating easier.

What aids are available for the bedroom?

For somebody with arthritis, the bedroom is a room of great importance for not only is it where much of the resting and exercising takes place, it is also the room in which dressing and grooming are performed. With suitable planning you could make this room into a type of command centre, where everything can be controlled from the one area.

It is now possible, for instance, to have the various electrical appliances in your house wired up to a control panel, which can operate many things from your bed. This can carry out such diverse activities as switching ovens on and off as well as electrically opening and closing doors, including the front and back doors – nowadays an increasingly important security consideration.

As well as this sophisticated form of control system, you should ensure that any essential communication equipment, such as the telephone, is conveniently situated together with necessary pencils and note pads where they are easily accessible.

Now, let us consider the bed. It is possible that your existing bed may already be perfectly suited to your condition and you may not have to change it. But do have a word with your doctor or physiotherapist to make sure that the bed you have *is* the best for your particular requirements. It may be too rigid or too unsupporting. If, for instance, you are advised that your bed should be more rigid and you are worried that your spouse may not wish to sleep in a more rigid bed there is a way around this problem. For it is possible to purchase a double bed that is rigid on one side and less rigid upon the other. Alternatively, a board can be placed beneath the mattress on your side only.

Sometimes if the bed is too low and presents difficulties when getting up, rather than buying a higher bed it is possible to increase the height of the bed by the use of bed-raisers.

If you find that, in the morning, stiffness is such a problem that it is difficult to raise yourself even to a sitting position, then you may find that a rope-ladder bed hoist is extremely helpful.

What aids are there to help me with dressing?

Make sure you have all your clothes easily to hand, and that they are readily accessible in drawers and shelves that are situated at convenient heights for you.

Now for the actual process of dressing. If you have problems doing up buttons there are two alternatives. You can either buy one of the many varieties of button-hooks that are available or, over the course of time, replace buttoned garments with clothing that may be fastened by zips. If you find that doing up a zip poses problems, it is possible to buy zippers that have a ring attached to the zip tag through which a thumb may be passed.

You may have problems in actually getting your clothes on. In this case a dressing stick will be invaluable.

For men, to save tying a tie, ready made-up ties are a useful alternative.

Often, the arthritic will have problems in bending down. Under these circumstances, a stocking aid allows socks and stockings to be drawn over the foot, long-handled shoe horns can help in putting shoes on, whilst special shoe removers perform the opposite task. Elastic shoe laces will also help in both respects.

What aids are available for the bathroom?

Of paramount importance, when considering how best to design a bathroom and the basic aids that should be included, is safety. Bathrooms can be dangerous places at the best of times, with water leaving many slippery surfaces. When such potential danger spots are exaggerated by the problems of manoeuvrability and stability that are all too common with arthritis it is even more important that great detail and attention be given to the bathroom and the fittings.

There are two pieces of equipment that are absolute necessities. The first of these is rails, in the form of hand-rails, 'grab bars' and bath rails, which should be fixed in places where they might obviously be needed in an emergency. The reason for these bars is self-evident, for, in the case of a potential fall, by holding onto them the arthritic sufferer will probably be able to avoid such serious injuries as a fractured hip or even a fractured skull.

The second piece of essential bathroom equipment is non-slip safety mats that can be placed at strategic spots where water might collect, such as by the basin or surrounding the bath. Bathmats that are nice and fluffy but with a tendency to slip on a bathroom's linoleum floor should be avoided.

I should now like to mention a few aids that you might find helpful.

Most modern lavatories, in keeping with what is considered to be 'fashionable bathroom fittings', are invariably low structures and even for those without arthritis can pose quite a problem when trying to sit down, and especially when wiping and arising again. These lavatories also tend to be put in the most confined spaces. Two things can be done to solve this problem. A raised lavatory seat can be fitted over the existing seat and hand rails placed to the side of the lavatory so that lowering yourself on to and raising yourself from the seat is made easier.

One of the greatest problems whilst on the lavatory can be wiping the anus. This can be greatly facilitated by the use of a lavatory paper holder. As to bathing and washing, getting in and out of baths can be helped by rails that attach around the taps and by which you can gently raise or lower yourself. Although you may not find too much difficulty in lowering yourself into the bath getting out of the bath will probably pose a greater problem.

The solution to this is to place a special seat in the bath. Although this may mean that you cannot get totally immersed in the water, it will at least allow you to manoeuvre in and around the bath more easily. Once in the bath there are a variety of implements that are available to help you wash. Taps are invariably difficult to turn on and off, so choose one of the many varieties of tap extensions that will make this task easier. Showers placed at inconvenient heights can be modified to the height that suits you or probably better still, can be designed to be hand-held. Other useful aids are special soap-holders and toothpaste-dispensers, and long-handled washing aids to help you wash extremities that you would not normally be able to reach.

As far as cleaning teeth is concerned, either an electric tooth brush or a tooth brush with an enlarged handle can be of benefit. Similarly razors, combs and hairbrushes will be much easier to manipulate if they have specially enlarged handles. If you encounter difficulties in grooming hair on the back of your head, combs and brushes with extended handles will overcome this problem.

What about the living room?

Consider how you spend most of your time. Do you like watching television, for instance? If so, do ensure that you have a remote control. This may involve a bit more expense but, in the long run, it is very worthwhile.

Consider also the chair in which you are going to be sitting. There is no need to go and buy a special orthopaedic chair – just see how you can modify the shape of your existing chair by the judicious use of cushions to best support your affected parts. Remember, if the chair is too comfortable, it is probably not doing your back too much good.

I realize that I have only touched upon a few aspects of ways in which you can improve the architecture of your home, to best suit your arthritic needs. I can only emphasize, once again, that you sit down, think your specific problems through and discuss the various solutions, always keeping safety aspects at the top of your list. Do not allow yourself to feel that the most expensive solution is always the best.

Finally, if moving to a new home, before deciding to move, look at it from the viewpoint of your arthritic needs. Although it may be your dream house, the house that you have always wanted to have, it may present you with insuperable problems when you actually come to live in it and have to adapt it to your particular problems.

What other aids can be used in the house?

As far as cleaning is concerned, long handles are probably the 'order of the day'. But this need not involve going out and buying special implements. You can simply modify your existing handles. If you are confined to a wheelchair, shortening these handles can make these chores easier.

Self-propelled vacuum cleaners take away the strain of pushing as do the very lightweight sweepers.

Electric plugs can be purchased with handles on them and specially adapted 'dialling sticks' can make phone dialling much easier although, in this respect, you may find button phones easier to use.

To save having to reach to pick things up, especially off the floor, all sorts of reachers are also available.

Doors and other keys can be fitted with enlarged handles as can pens and pencils, and a variety of non-slip surfaces and epoxy compounds that can be affixed to most household articles is also available.

What aids are available for when I go out?

If you are a passenger in a car the passenger seat can be modified so that it swivels, allowing ease of access. There are also a variety of aids that can help in getting from a wheelchair into a car. Special car door openers are also available, for opening car doors.

When out shopping, a shopping trolley is a good idea and trolleys which also double up as ambulatory aids are especially useful.

Do remember, at all times, that pavements are always a potential hazard due to their unevenness and that shop floors cleaned for hygienic purposes can be very slippery.

Gardening is a hobby of mine. Can I still do it if I have arthritis?

In the main, if pursued judiciously, gardening can be both an extremely good form of exercise and an eminently satisfying and rewarding activity. It is an area of activity which, if planned through properly, can be pursued with success even though the arthritic sufferer may be physicially quite restricted. Addresses of organizations that can give helpful advice are given on p.146. However, I should just like to mention some basic principles that you might like to bear in mind before looking at the large variety of ideas and implements that are available to help the arthritic sufferer in the garden.

Let us start with the back and back-related problems. This doesn't just apply to those with an arthritic back problem. Many back problems can start in the garden, particularly through digging in heavy, clay soils.

So, a few basic rules.

Throughout the digging action try not to bend your back. Keeping a rigidly straight back, however, may be counter-productive and may even put unnecessary strain on certain muscle groups. Reach a sensible compromise, therefore, keeping the bending to a minimum.

Make sure you use the right sort of spade. The essentials to look for are lightness in weight, ease of grip, length of handle and sharpness of the digging edge. When actually digging, as I mentioned when advising on lifting, use the knees and hips to exert the necessary force rather than allowing the back joints to take the strain.

Another area where this advice is paramount is in the use of wheelbarrows. When using a wheelbarrow, do not overload it. In the long run you will put less stress on your joints by making more frequent trips with it only half-full than by a single or a few heavily laden journeys. This principle of doing tasks in the garden in measured, small and easily achievable steps is a good general working rule.

Now, some more specific tips on equipment and other ways of making certain gardening tasks easier. As a general guideline, remember that stainless steel tools often penetrate soil more easily. Also, remember that the handles of most tools are available in forms that can be adapted to compensate for the majority of hand disabilities. Such handles fall into two main groups: the extension type of handle that allows for working from the sitting or standing position when bending is difficult or impossible, and the type of handle that, in effect, enlarges the handle of existing tools.

In this respect, it is very important to make use of what you already have. If you find that you are having problems holding a trowel, just take some old material and bind it about the trowel's handle and you will almost certainly find that it is very much easier to grip. Alternatively, there are commercially available foam or plastic materials that can be applied to the handles of most gardening tools.

When both hoeing and raking, use the lightest possible implements with the longest possible handles or extensions if necessary.

Just because you may find yourself confined to a wheelchair does not mean to say that you cannot perform many of gardening's more pleasurable tasks as long as you adopt certain measures. When working in the greenhouse, ensure that all working surfaces are at the optimum height for you. Also, be careful when moving heavy objects like flower pots from shelves – they are often heavier than you expect when you are in a sitting position and are usually more difficult to control.

You may find that constantly working at normal ground level becomes tiring. In this case, have you thought of having some of your flower beds raised so that they are at a more acceptable and convenient height for you to work at?

When working from a wheelchair the lightest tools possible with the most convenient extensions are all-important for with such simple labour saving devices what can be a gardening chore can turn into a gardening delight. Before purchasing anything, however, do remember to try it out. Just because it is expensive does not mean to say that it is necessarily for you.

Glossaries &
Useful Addresses

Glossary of Terms

Abduction   The movement of a limb away from the midline of the body.

Acetabulum   The socket in the hip bone into which the head of the femur (thigh bone) fits.

Acromegaly   A condition in which the bones and soft tissues become enlarged as a result of the excess production of growth hormone.

Acupuncture   The insertion of needles on specific skin meridians in order to alleviate, or cure disease, or anaesthetize.

Adduction   The movement of a limb towards the midline of the body.

Agglutination Test   A chemical test to reveal the presence of antibodies in bodily fluids.

Anaemia   A relative deficiency of haemoglobin-containing red cells.

Analgesic   A pain-killing drug.

Ankylosis   Immobility of a joint due to replacement of normal joint tissue by fibrous tissue.

Antibody   An agent of the body's defence system, produced to fight inflection or substances detected as being foreign.

Antigen   A substance that the body's immune system detects as being foreign to its tissues. Also called an allergen.

Arteritis   An inflammatory response occurring in the wall of an artery.

Arthralgia   Pain arising from a joint.

Arthrodesis   Surgical fusion of a joint resulting in joint immobilization and relief of joint pain.

Arthroplasty   The surgical remodelling or remoulding of a diseased joint.

Arthroscopy   The insertion of an instrument into a joint allowing the surgeon to inspect anatomical structures within the joint.

Arthrosis   Non-inflammatory joint disease.

Atrophy   Shrinkage or wasting of a tissue such as a muscle.

Auto-Immune   The word given to the defect in the body's immune system (white cells and antibodies) that causes the body to manufacture antibodies that attack the body's own tissue.

Bacteria   Single-celled, microscopic organisms responsible for bacterial infections.

Biopsy   The removal of a specimen piece of tissue for the purpose of diagnosis.

Bunion   A swelling on the first joint of the big toe as a result of inflammation.

Bursa   A small, fluid-filled sac found between tendons and bones, which allows the tendon to glide smoothly over the bone.

Bursitis   Inflammation occurring with a bursa.

Calcification   Deposition of calcium salts within a tissue.

Capsulectomy   Surgical removal of a joint capsule.

Cartilage   Fibrous connective tissue covering the ends of bones.

Cervical   Term used to describe the anatomical region of the neck.

Collagen   Chemically composed of protein, collagen is the main fibrous tissue responsible for the strength of a variety of tissues including ligaments and bones (collagen disease refers to pathological change in collagenous tissue).

Connective Tissue   These tissues have as their major chemical component, collagen (see above). It is a term sometimes used synonymously with collagenous tissue.

Contracture   The shrinkage or physical shortening of tissues such as tendons, ligaments and muscles.

Dermatitis   Inflammation of the skin.

Erosions   Crater-like hollows seen in bones at joint sites.

Extension   The movement of a joint into a straight position.

Fascitis   Inflammation of the fibrous tissue which surrounds and lies between muscle groups.

Fibroblasts   Cells responsible for the construction of the connective tissues of the body.

Fibrositis   A non-specific term used to describe inflammation, pain and stiffness in general.

Flexion   The bending of a joint.

Gout   A condition in which there are raised levels of uric acid in the body. High levels of uric acid crystals in joints gives rise to gouty arthritis.

Haemarthrosis   A joint in which there has been bleeding.

Haemoglobin   A protein carried by red blood cells responsible for the carriage and exchange of oxygen and carbon dioxide.

Haemophilia   A deficiency of factor VIII, a blood clotting factor, resulting in a tendency to bleed, especially into joints.

Hamstrings   The tendons of the muscles that run down the back of the leg to the knee.

Heberden's Nodes   Bony outcrops of the finger joints which are often seen in osteoarthritis.

Intervertebral Disc   Connective tissue separating vertebrae.

Isometric Exercise   Muscular contraction without joint movement.

Kyphosis   A deformity of the spine resulting in a forwards curvature.

Ligaments   Strong bands of connective tissue that hold the parts of the skeleton in the correct alignment.

Lordosis   Forward curvature in the lower back.

Lumbago   A non-specific term indicating pain in the lower back.

Lumbar   Term used to describe the anatomical region of the lower back.

Lymphocyte   A variety of white cell which plays an integral part in the body's immune system.

Musculoskeletal   A term referring to both muscle and bone.

Myalgia   Pain arising from within muscle.

Myelogram   A radiological procedure involving the introduction of radio opaque material into the cerebro-spinal fluid that surrounds the spinal cord.

Myopathy   A weakness of muscle.

Myositis   Inflammation of muscle.

Nodule   A non-specific term referring to a lump just beneath the surface of the skin.

Osteomalacia   Loss of the mineral content of bone resulting in bone weakness.

Osteomyelitis   Infection or inflammation of the bone.

Osteophytes   Outgrowth from bone seen in any joint affected by osteoarthritis.

Osteoporosis   A loss of the protein component of bones resulting in the thinning of the bones.

Osteotomy   A surgical incision into bone.

Pannus   Vascularization of the synovial membrane seen in rheumatoid arthritis.

Periosteum   A fibrous tissue that lines bones.

Phlebitis   Inflammation in the wall of a vein.

Polyarteritis   Inflammation in a number of arteries.

Prosthesis   An artificial substitute for an anatomical structure.

Psoriasis   A chronic inflammatory skin condition that waxes and wanes; sometimes responsible for arthritis.

Raynaud's Disease   A circulatory disease in which the blood vessels supplying the fingers and toes suddenly contract, reducing blood flow to these areas. This results in pallor, coldness and diminished sensation.

Rheumatoid Factor   An antibody often found in the tissues of those suffering with rheumatoid arthritis.

Sacro-iliac Joint   The joint between the hip bones and the lower part of the spine.

Scleroderma   A condition characterized by hardening and thickening of the skin due to a chronic inflammatory process occurring with ithe connective tissues of the skin.

Scoliosis   A deformity of the spine resulting in a sideways curve of the vertebrae.

Spondylitis   Inflammation occurring in the joints of the spine.

Spondylosis   Degenerative changes occurring within the spinal column specifically in the area of the intervertebral discs.

Supination   The outward rotation of the arm resulting in the palm facing upwards.

Synovectomy   Surgical removal of the synovial membrane.

Synovial Fluid   The lubricating fluid found within synovial joints.

Synovial Joint   A joint lined by a synovial membrane.

Synovial Membrane   A specialized, thin sheet of tissue that is responsible for the secretion of synovial fluid both in synovial joints, in bursas and in the sheaths that surround tendons.

Systemic Lupus Erythematosus   An inflammatory disease of the small blood vessels that supply many structures of the body such as the kidneys, the skin, the lungs and the joints.

Tendon   A connective tissue made up of collagen that allows muscles to be attached to bone.

Tendonitis   Inflammation of a tendon.

Tenosynovitis   An inflammation of the synovial membrane surrounding a tendon.

Tenotomy   The surgical division of a tendon.

Tophi   Large collections of uric acid crystals, often seen in the hands and feet of gout sufferers.

Traction   A pulling force, the purpose of which is to relieve pressure on a joint.

Trans-cutaneous Nerve Stimulation   An electrical means of pain relief.

Ultrasound   High frequency sound waves used to relieve inflammation.

Uric acid   A normal constituent of blood but which, if found in raised levels, can be responsible for gout.

Valgus Deformity   A deformity resulting in outward displacement from the body; an example being bow legs.

Vasculitis   Inflammation of blood vessels.

Vertebrae   The bones which makes up the spinal column.

Xerostomia   A dry sensation of the month.

Drug Glossary

ALLOPURINOL
ADMINISTRATION Oral.
USES Reduction of uric acid levels.
POSSIBLE SIDE-EFFECTS Allergic skin reactions; gastro-intestinal upsets.

ASPIRIN
ADMINISTRATION Oral.
USES Pain killing; anti-inflammatory. Used in both rheumatoid arthritis and osteoarthritis.
POSSIBLE SIDE-EFFECTS Stomach and duodenal ulceration; gastro-intestinal upsets; ringing in the ears; episodes of imbalance; allergic reactions; adversely affects anticoagulant therapy.

CHLOROQUINE
ADMINISTRATION Oral
USES Anti-inflammatory.
POSSIBLE SIDE-EFFECTS The main problem is damage to the eye – regular eye examinations are, therefore, mandatory. Other problems are damage to both the kidneys and the liver; gastro-intestinal upsets; allergic skin reactions; harmful effects on blood cells.

CODEINE PHOSPHATE
ADMINISTRATION Oral.
USES Pain relief.
POSSIBLE SIDE-EFFECTS Constipation; nausea; not recommended with alcohol.

COLCHICINE
ADMINISTRATION Oral.
USES Reduces joint inflammation.
POSSIBLE SIDE-EFFECTS Gastro-intestinal upsets; allergic skin reactions.

FENBUFEN
ADMINISTRATION Oral.
USES Anti-inflammatory.
POSSIBLE SIDE-EFFECTS Similar to ibuprofen but is said to cause less gastro-intestinal disturbance.

HYDROCORTISONE ACETATE
ADMINISTRATION Injection into site of pain.
USES Anti-inflammatory.
POSSIBLE SIDE-EFFECTS Encouragement of local or systemic infection; damage and weakening of structures in local area such as muscle and tendon if frequently repeated.

IBUPROFEN
ADMINISTRATION Oral.
USES Anti-inflammatory.
POSSIBLE SIDE-EFFECTS Normally minimal although can cause gastro-intestinal upset and, rarely, allergic skin rashes.

INDOMENTHACIN
ADMINISTRATION Oral/Suppository.
USES Anti-inflammatory.
POSSIBLE SIDE-EFFECTS Can cause drowsiness; can be responsible for allergic symptoms such as asthma; gastro-intestinal disturbances including peptic ulceration; headaches together with feelings of light-headedness and anaemia; prolonged use can affect the eyes.

KETOPROFEN
ADMINISTRATION Oral.
USES Mild anti-inflammatory.
POSSIBLE SIDE-EFFECTS Similar to ibuprofen (see above).

MEFANAMIC ACID
ADMINISTRATION Oral.
USES Mainly pain relief with some anti-inflammatory action.
POSSIBLE SIDE-EFFECTS Diarrhoea and anaemia.

NAPROXEN
ADMINISTRATION Oral Suppository.
USES Mainly anti-inflammatory though with mild pain-killing properties.
POSSIBLE SIDE-EFFECTS Normally minimal; can cause gastro-intestinal upsets and allergic reactions; sometimes ringing in the ear is heard.

PARACETAMOL
ADMINISTRATION Oral.
USES Pain relief.
POSSIBLE SIDE-EFFECTS Normally well-tolerated; excessive intake can result in liver damage.

PENICILLAMINE
ADMINISTRATION Oral.
USES Disease-modifying.
POSSIBLE SIDE-EFFECTS Damage to blood cells; damage to the kidney; allergic reactions; gastro-intestinal upsets.

PHENYLBUTAZONE
ADMINISTRATION Oral.
USES Anti-inflammatory.
POSSIBLE SIDE-EFFECTS This drug has now been withdrawn from general use because it can cause an acute reduction in production of the white cells of the blood, leaving the patient unable to fight off infection. It is now only used by rheumatologists under strict clinical control.

PIROXICAM
ADMINISTRATION Oral Suppository.
USES Anti-inflammatory.
POSSIBLE SIDE-EFFECTS Similar to ibuprofen.

PREDNISOLONE
ADMINISTRATION Oral/Intramuscular/Intravenous.
USES Anti-inflammatory.
POSSIBLE SIDE-EFFECTS Growth suppression in children; raised blood pressure; may cause diabetes and osteoporosis; psychiatric conditions such as depression; gastro-intestinal upsets including peptic ulcerations masking of underlying infection; suppression of the adrenal gland.

PROBENECID
ADMINISTRATION Oral.
USES Reduction of uric acid levels.
POSSIBLE SIDE-EFFECTS Normally well tolerated: gastro-intestinal upsets; occasional damage to kidney, liver and bone marrow.

SODIUM AUROTHIOMALATE
ADMINISTRATION Intramuscular.
USES Disease-modifying.
POSSIBLE SIDE-EFFECTS Allergic responses; renal damage; suppression of bone marrow.

Useful Addresses

Arthritis and Rheumatism Council
41 Eagle Street
London WC1
01 405 8572

Arthritis Care
6 Grosvenor Crescent
London SW1 7ER
01 235 0902

The Back Pain Association
Park House
31-33 Park Road
Teddington
Middlesex TW11 0AB
01 977 5474

British Society for Rheumatology
41 Eagle Street
London WC1
01 405 8572

Royal Association for Disability and Rehabilitation
25 Mortimer Street
London W1N 8AB
01 637 5400

Central Council for the Disabled
This has been amalgamated into the Royal Association for Disability and Rehabilitation (see above)

Index

Index

prognosis 57, 58
splinting joints 90
symptoms 57
treatment 62, 67, 72, 90
and use of steroids 67, 70

K
Ketoprofen 65, 146
Keys 135
Kidneys, effects on 24, 25
Kitchen, organizing the 124, 129-31
Knee joints 14
    bursitis in (housemaid's knee) 51
    osteoarthritis in 15, 25
    pseudogout in 31
    rheumatoid arthritis in 100-1
    surgical operation on 101-2
Knives 131
Kyphosis 142

L
Lavatory, aids to using the 133-4
Legs:
    claudication of 54
    cramp in 53-4, 55
    pain due to slipped disc 34
    pain in 54-5, 104
    swollen 49-50
Lifting heavy objects 81, 105-6
Ligaments 36, 142
Lighting in the home 129
Locks, security 129
Lordosis 142
Lumbago 143
Lumps under skin 50
Lungs, effects on 24, 25
Lymph glands, enlarged 18, 42, 56
Lymphocytes 143

M
Malaria, drugs for 74
Markers, chemical 36, 37

Massage 90
Mats 128, 133
Mattresses 80, 105, 106
Meals:
    cooking 124, 129-31
    eating aids 131
Mechanical aids 126-8
    for housework 135
    in the kitchen 130-1
    safety aspects 126-7
Mefanamic acid 146
Menopause, the 49
Mental capacity 20-1
Meridians 117
Metatarsalgia 83-4
Morning stiffness 17, 24, 80
Motivation, lack of 110
Moving house 135
Mugs, double-handled 131
Myalgia 143
Myelogram 143
Myocarditis 67
Myopathy 71
Myositis 143

N
Naproxen 65, 146
Neck pain:
    medical causes of 106
    psychological causes of 107-8
    and use of collars 108-9
Nerves:
    impairment of blood supply to 23
    trapped 55, *see also* Carpal tunnel syndrome
Nerve stimulation, transcutaneous electrical 121
Nodules 50, 143
Non-steroidal anti-inflammatory drugs (NSAIDs) 62, 64, 66, 71

O
Obesity: and arthritis of the hip